RANSOMING
THE MIND

RANSOMING THE MIND

An Integration of Yoga and Modern Therapy

Charles T. Bates

Foreword by Rudolph M. Ballentine, M.D.

YES International, Publishers
St. Paul, Minnesota

The author is sensitive to the absence of a non-specific gender designator in English. Those temporary solutions occasionally used by enlightened writers are, at best, awkward. For the sake of style and ease in reading, the traditional masculine pronouns have been used in this book. It is hoped that the literary, academic and philosophical communities will soon take the lead in creating a pronoun that singularly stands for both sexes.

RANSOMING THE MIND. Copyright 1986 by Charles T. Bates. All rights reserved. No part of this book may be used or reproduced in any manner whatsoever without written permission except in the case of brief quotations embodied in critical articles and reviews. For information address YES International, 449 Portland Avenue, St. Paul, Minnesota 55102.

LC: 86-50084
ISBN: 0-936663-00-6

Printed in the United States of America

Contents

Foreword   *vii*

Preface   *xi*

Acknowledgements   *xv*

What Is Therapy?   1

What Is Yoga?   15

The Addiction Process   31

Addiction: The Yoga Parallel   49

The Mind in Yoga   71

Steps to Transformation   87

Diet   107

Body Work   123

Yoga Postures   149

Relaxation   263

Breathing   283

Meditation   313

Foreword

Modern society is seriously affected by an epidemic. It is chemical dependency. The creativity and promise of young people is being lost in the isolation and confusion of drug experiences. The wisdom of maturity is dulled and eventually destroyed by alcohol. There is hardly a family untouched by drug problems today. Yet modern physicians and psychiatrists have been largely unsuccessful in their attempts to remedy this serious problem. Many therapies and treatment programs have been devised and implemented, but the sad truth is that the failure rate is staggering. Even in those cases when initial success seems apparent, follow-up shows that recidivism is high.

To cope with this serious problem, modern man must look deep into his attitudes and habit patterns to understand what makes him susceptible to the process of addiction. What is needed is a way of scrutinizing modern values and approaches to life. Yet the very scientists and therapists who should help with the solution are so caught up in the prevailing values and attitudes that they are unable to step free of them to discern the fundamental basis of the problem. Therefore the damage done by chemical dependency continues. In such a dilemma, bringing to bear a different perspective—one uncolored and unaffected by modern life and current thinking—can help to clear the air and bring to light the weaknesses upon which chemical dependency preys.

The perennial psychology of the ancient sages has much to say about the basis of suffering in mankind and its tendency to withdraw into the comforts of an addictive drug. This perspective, brought into the treatment of chemical dependency, has yielded astonishing results.

Skilled in the principles and traditions of yoga science, Charles Bates designed an experimental program that applied yogic techniques to the re-education and reawakening of creativity in several groups of young people who had been seriously affected by their involvement with drugs. The results were not only interesting, they were like a breath of fresh air in a field long accustomed to disappointments and bad news. The principles and practice of yoga provided a means of awakening a sense of exploration and self-discovery in those who were involved. Those who participated in his programs over the years have found their way out of chemical dependency into productive and satisfying lives.

In his innovative book, Charles Bates discusses the application of yoga psychology and yoga-oriented therapy to the treatment of chemical dependency. He offers practical and common-sensical concepts as well as a repertoire of therapeutic techniques that have been tested in his work and found to be useful and effective.

The pointers given on the specific use of yoga postures, relaxation, breathing techniques, and the application of the meditative attitude to dealing with such psychological problems as those involved in chemical dependency will be useful not only to the clinician who works in this area, but to the average person who must of necessity deal with his own tendency toward addictions of all sorts, and who must work through those to rediscover himself and reclaim his birthright to creativity and self-discovery.

RUDOLPH M. BALLENTINE, M.D.

Director, Combined Therapy Program
Himalayan Inernational Institute

Preface

Over the years and under the guidance of my teacher, Sri Swami Rama of the Himalayas, it has been my privilege to develop and implement an application of classical yoga to modern therapy. At the various treatment centers and hospitals at which I have worked, I designed programs which proved to be very successful. It was not my intention to install yoga as a replacement to conventional therapeutic approaches, but to design programs to complement the treatment models already in place.

Several physicians, counselors, therapists, and yoga teachers among my colleagues asked if it was possible to set these programs into book form to serve as a manual for therapists. They hoped that it would be possible for the many treatment centers across the country to benefit from this integration of yoga and modern therapy. *Ransoming the Mind* is an attempt to that end.

In the course of writing this book, my experiences and observations of some yoga masters have been added to show their methods of eliciting transformation in close students. I have been amazed and delighted by what I saw, and I hope I have been able to convey some of the essence of their great skill within these pages.

I have taken the liberty of commenting upon my

observations of the application of therapy in view of the yoga paradigm for health, and have made some parallels between current therapy and yoga as it is used in its preliminary stages for clearing psychological obstacles.

A chapter on the addiction process has been included to show how one becomes consumed by an agent outside of oneself—chemical dependency. A chapter on how one is consumed by an agent inside of oneself—the inner need for psychological safety—is paralleled. Comments on the centuries-old methods of self-unfoldment from the perspective of an initiator of transformation are given with the suggestion that the initiator be very clear that first, he is working with himself more than with the client, and second, he is not there to tell the client what to do, but only to offer greater and clearer choices in how to be.

The classical yoga paradigm is a holistic one. It holds with the ancient realization that transformation of a human being must be addressed on all levels and dimensions. We are not only an intellect, as the term "psychology" implies. In the study of human development more than the psyche impacts our growth. The body can assist or impede development. As a result, I have devoted a section to transformation work from the body's perspective giving detailed programs and explanations in the yoga postures. A section on diet is also included consistent with the ever-increasing evidence that we really are what we eat. Yogic sages have long implemented the powerful dynamic of the breath, and so I have devoted a section to breathing as it is related to the therapeutic paradigm. The use of relaxation in therapy is included with the detailed instructions and techniques of classical relaxation methods. Meditation as a technique of the quiet observation of life is explained and outlined in what I hope is an easily understandable process.

All in all my intention is that the reader will have in his hands a manual that will allow him to implement a critical, clear, and safe application of yoga techniques from its therapeutic perspective and at the same time be in the partnership of learning along with the people he is teaching.

My offering to yoga teachers is that they deliver the application of this book to their students in light of health rather than dysfunction. The techniques have originated from years of study and guidance with my teacher as well as my observation of other yogic adepts, some very powerful communicators, and my experience in therapeutic communities across the country using Western psychological techniques.

May all those in the helping professions benefit from the ideas offered in *Ransoming the Mind*.

CHARLES BATES

Acknowledge-
ments

The author would like to acknowledge the enormous amount of patience and love of his teacher, Sri Swami Rama, in waiting so long for this book to appear. There would be no book were it not for his view of the inner workings of the mind imparted to me in ways that appeared at times to border on the magical. Any mistranslation of that view is my error and does not belong to the tradition.

Secondly, I would like to acknowledge Theresa King O'Brien, who is next in line for the responsibility for this book. It was her commitment that inspired me to be disciplined. She has pulled the book out of me and has sat with me through many hours of dictation, re-writing, editing, and typing. The rough threads of my thoughts have been woven by her into a fabric suitable for wear.

I would also like to thank Horst Rechelbacher, president of the Aveda Corporation based in Minneapolis, for lending his photography staff, particularly Sandy Rumreich, who took all the photos in the hatha yoga section. Many thanks to my student, Dr. Gordon May-field, of Mayfield Chiropractic and Holistic Health Care Center in St. Paul, for performing the yoga postures.

I am grateful to all the writers and workshop leaders whose reflections and expertise have contributed over the years to my learning.

Finally I would like to thank my colleague and friend, Dr. Justin O'Brien, for his well-chosen words and support, as well as his gift of the book's title.

1
What Is
Therapy?

Over past centuries the care for the soul of man
has been under the custodianship of the priestly order.
It was the priest's role in the human family to chart
salvation, interpret the dimensions of the psyche, give
guidelines that were designed to correct deviations
from the path, and dispel the darkness in the mind
of man. The twentieth century, however, has seen
an interesting shift of the primary responsibility for
guiding the development of the psyche from the priests
to another order—that of the psychiatrist, the therapist,
the counselor.

Therapy is a corrective model designed to approach and solve a behavior that is interpreted as dysfunctional. This model presupposes that the organism is physiologically or psychologically out of ease to the extent that assistance must be given to return the organism to a perceived balance. Therapy appears to presuppose a norm, and when individuals act psychologically outside of that norm, either in their own opinion or in the opinion of others, efforts are made to assist them (or sometimes force them) back within an acceptable framework ascertained by the therapist, or in few cases, by the client himself.

In a sense the dysfunction of the psyche is a creation of therapy. I do not mean to say that there are not psychological dysfunctions, but that the types of dysfunction observed are dependent upon the parameters of therapeutics, more specifically, on the therapist. Therapy is based on the presupposition of disease. The context by which exploration into disease is advanced is then woven out of a fabric of discord with the intent of re-establishing accord.

The question is, Is it humanly possible to create health out of a disease model? What criteria does one establish to determine when health comes into existence? Health, some say, is the absence of disease. I wonder if it is as cut and dried as that. I wonder if in the case of a lack of disease health is the only other possibility that can show up. Is it accurate to define a state by the absence of its absence? The proposal here is that the context from which questions arise should also be investigated to expose the possibility of fallacy in our presuppositions and/or process. This is so because there may be more to the question than what the questioner brings to the issue. We can only pursue removing what we interpret needs removing.

In the course of the development of modern therapy, a number of schools of thought have emerged and are in use to achieve therapeutic goals. The goals found to be satisfied by the therapist are by nature of their invention structured within the context of their creation. Modern psychology is young on the scene of mind care. The ethics and exploration of mental health in our time is visibly and invisibly subjective and may be colored with historical, unexamined notions.

Various schools of thought have discovered diverse dimensions of the human psyche and have targeted their exploration via the dictates of their particular discovery. It is somewhat like the story of the blind men who each encountered a different part of an elephant's body. Each one described the elephant according to the sensory data he was capable of gathering and interpreting. Each then generalized his discovery to describe the entire elephant and every other elephant.

Although the founders of many of the schools of psychology did not believe their approach to be a complete one, therapy is, generally speaking, applied as if the approach of a school accurately delineates the human condition and has the perception of the norm. Each school, then, approaches personal development from a different direction. Let us take a brief look at some of the major schools influencing therapy today.

In the **Behavioral** school of thought behavior is considered to be based on conditioned reflex. Behaviorists see the adult personality as a superimposition of many instances of conditioning upon a basic set of innate behavior patterns. From a behavioral perspective personality consists of patterns of learned behavior. This learning or conditioning can be based on either associating a new stimulus with an old one or by rewarding, that is, reinforcing, a behavior after it occurs. These two types of learning are known respectively as classical and operant conditioning, and are the means by which all behavior is generated. Behaviorists consider that biology dictates the evolution that we call humankind. The mind has its source in biology and only observable behavior that can be objectively measured is the basis for science. Subjective states which cannot be externally observed and measured do not meet the cirteria for satisfactory scientific inquiry into human behavior. This premise appears to structure reality as existing within the framework of currently observable, measureable phenomenon that can be replicated.

Psychoanalysis finds its source of thought in the acknowledgement of an unconscious dimension to the human mind. Freudian psychoanalysis aims at exploring unconscious conflict which results from the experiences in infancy and childhood. In psychoanalysis humans are viewed as needing to resolve conflicting unconscious drives and reconcile the components of these drives. Because of unconscious urges interfacing with conscious moral demands, defense mechanisms have developed. Therapy is directed at the production of successful behavior through the redirection of these primal unconscious desires.

The **Jungian** approach acknowledges that there is a subjective reality to the human mind that is outside of conscious awareness. Analysis of the unconscious material through interpretation of dreams and free association are two techniques used to explore this unconscious mind. This system examines the existence of universal principles or archetypes as being significant factors in the expression of human development. Hypnosis has also been used as a technique to reaccess inaccessable and repressed information stored outside of conscious awareness.

The **Adlerian** approach proposes that man is a social animal that has the ability to adapt to psychological environments. In order to successfully do this he must be able to free himself from feelings of inadequacy and the resulting compulsive behavior to eliminate those feelings of inferiority. If he is not successful, he will be chasing phantoms that disappear like smoke when embraced. This behavior is viewed as neurotic. The normal human being has the same feeling of inadequacy, but phantoms prove to have practical value as guide-posts and do not imprison the seeker on a quest of mirages.

The school of thought founded by Karen **Horney** closely parallels an ancient system within the Buddhist structure called the five *skandhas* (see page 57-60.). Horney states that human beings, in coping with an environment that seems to threaten their individuality, view themselves as isolated and develop neurotic mechanisms to cope with that environment. They become the victims of compulsive urges of self-preservation and employ aggression, submission, and detachment to maintain their identity. They then find themselves imprisoned within the walls of their neurotic solutions and tendencies.

The theory of **Gestalt** comes from the German word for "pattern." For the Gestaltist the whole pattern or context of an experience is more important than its individual parts. Behavior is associated with patterns in one's own personal history. These pattterns stem from urges associated with our infancy and childhood, desires associated with our young adulthood, and desires associated with our mature parental self. For instance, when in the presence of an authoritarian figure, a thirty-five-year-old may respond out of a twelve-year-old's pattern of powerlessness and defiance generated in childhood. At any given time one of these desires will be dominant and appeal must be made to the various parts for transformation. Conversation is then set up by the therapist, a peer, or the subject himself to explore the source of the dysfunction.

The **Rogerian** therapist acknowledges and accepts the behavior of the client totally and unconditionally, regardless of its content. The acceptance of one human being for another is considered the fertile soil for self-love out of which will grow a sense of self-worth and personal acknowledgement. The system affirms that it is from this humanness and respect of self that a productive member of our society will flower.

Reality therapy explores personal development totally by focusing on the present, stating basically that any transformation that is to take place, takes place in the present and that focusing on the past purely serves to perpetuate unwanted historical behavior. Transformation is now, and now is what the mature being is to explore.

The last school that I would like to discuss is Abraham **Maslow's** theory. His theories were developed from working with people who felt themselves to be successful in life and were not considered socially dysfunctional. His approach was directed at people who were secure and were seeking what he called self-actualization. The objective for the therapist was to assist people in this direction and in the process coach them in becoming more satisfied with themselves. This approach to human development shares elements with the yogic model, as do certain dimensions of the other schools mentioned above, as we shall see in the following chapters.

Applications to bring about the goals of these various therapies as well as conditions that would satisfy the therapist are varied. The techniques range from changing only conscious behavior to accessing and negotiating alternate behaviors on an other-than-conscious level. Some approaches used by therapists are mentioned below.

Confrontive type therapies directly approach the conscious mind with what is considered inappropriate behavior. Responsibility for "acting out" inappropriately is laid directly upon the individual. This is thought to produce a mature, thoughtful member of society.

In the **Group Dynamics** approach to therapy the therapist engages a number of clients simultaneously. He and the other clients focus on one of the clients, assisting him to become aware of behavior that they as a group see clearly but that is out of the awareness of the person with whom they are working. This person will also reveal to the group those secrets that are outside of the group's awareness about his personal source of motivation. Through a combination of that which is known by everyone, that which is known only to the individual client, and that which is known by others but not by the client, a quality of self-knowledge will develop whereby the client will become more aware of that which is unknown to himself and to others. The therapeutic outcomes of this therapy also seek to intensify the emotional spectrum, for it is felt that the client is not aware of the emotional basis of his behavior or has systematically repressed his emotions to the point where he is no longer aware of their movement. He is encouraged to realize that feelings are valid pieces of data and must be incorporated in the cognition and structuring of reality.

Psychoanalysis seeks to sublimate emotional behavior that is considered to produce neuroses. The individual client is encouraged to become conscious of defenses such as repression, denial, and projection. He is also encouraged to become aware of complexes such as the oedipus complex, narcisscism, or the electra complex, whose source lies in the unconscious mind but the acting out of which violates his current values.

Bioenergetics explores how the body stores defenses by armoring itself against unwanted memories of feelings and anticipated reoccurance of unwanted stimulation. The body does this by stiffening itself against experiencing events kinestetically. Portions of the body are subjectively targeted as the receptor and experiencer of particular emotions. Once targeted and identified as an area in need of defense, unconscious strategies are employed, such as rigidity, enervation, or the total dropping out of awareness of the body part. Techniques to fatigue or manipulate the defensive mechanism are employed to introduce the opportunity to re-experience that which has been purposefully put out of awareness.

One thing to be considered is that most contemporary psychotherapy is based on a communication of

words between the therapist and the client. The very
fact that the contextual structure is communicated by
way of words of necessity creates a boundary that
has most probably not been considered and is thus
invisible to most practitioners. I wonder what kind of
interesting and delightful new outcomes could be
invented in addition to, and along with, contemporary
techniques if exploration was also taken in the direction of the expansion of sensory awareness—an
expansion that included communication that was outside of the medium delineated by words. Some
approaches that are exploring transcending this boundary are bioenergetics, rolfing, and breathing therapy.

Words are the interpretation of the speaker. Words
are the interpretation of the listener. Granted, we are
currently bound to language. The client speaks his
interpretation; the therapist listens through his interpretation. The therapist then responds through his
interpretation and the client listens again through his
interpretation. The interpretation is the limit, the
self-imposed limit and directional vehicle of the therapeutic encounter.

The setting of the circumstance is that the client
has a presenting problem. Or should we also add that
the set of circumstances is that the therapist is there
with the intention of encountering the set called problems? The fact that a client has been said to "have a
problem" comes out of the context, or fabric, of
problems. Do problems beget solutions or do they
beget their own kind? Problems beget problems.
Humans beget humans. Elm seeds beget elm trees.
Consider the possibility that problems cannot beget
solutions due to the fact that solutions do not exist

inside of the set called problems. This idea is expressed well by the French: *Plus ça change, plus c'est la même chose.** When one explores a paradigm that which is yeilded is that which is of the paradigm.

When a therapist is involved with a client, there is a presupposition that the client has a problem. The premise in which therapy is involved is in identifying problems. In this sense, therapy is the victim of its creation. It was created out of the need to address psychological dysfunction. As a result the child being born from the parent carries the presuppositions or geneological characteristics of the parents. The child in this case is psychological therapy, and the parents are psychological problems. This is a subtle issue that must be understood. I will give a case in point.

A young married couple came to me to get my view of their marriage. The young man so wanted the relationship to work that he listed his set of "problems" and said that he would do anything to correct himself so that the relationship could be reconciled. Our first work together was to explore the way he organized reality. As long as he was functioning in the domain or context of problems, he would continue, as he had been for the past seven years of marriage and the past twenty-four years of life, to have problems. The way he spoke of his "problems" invalidated almost his entire life up to that point. He was saying "The way I have done it in the past is wrong and now I want to do it right. In doing that I can be a better person."

This presupposes to me that there is someone inside of him who is intentionally doing wrong things

---

* "The more things change, the more they remain the same."

WHAT IS THERAPY?   11

to sabotage his life, and if he were only able to stop or correct that someone, things would be O.K. I introduced what was from my view a more constructive representation to the young man that also acknowledged the need he felt for transformation.

We first validated his past behavior as the best he knew how to do at the time he did it. Manipulating his mother to get out of work, not being responsible to other human beings, and behaving immaturely when he didn't get his way were agreements that he and his mother had established as appropriate. They worked with his mother from infancy on to the present, and had worked with his wife, because he had very carefully chosen someone who was willing to establish the same kind of agreements he had with his mother. That is, they had worked with his wife until three months prior to our meeting. His wife stated that she was annoyed by his lack of commitment and immaturity and wanted to leave the relationship. The young man, panic stricken, said that he was willing to do whatever necessary to please his wife so that she would stay.

He was so caught in his problems that he didn't know he was using old "problematic" behavior which would continue to generate the status quo. His old strategy was that whenever he would receive disapproval from his mother, he would, for the shortest time necessary, acquiesce until he saw her satisfied. When he felt the time was right, he would then return to his old patterns of behavior. He was now employing the same strategy with his wife. His emphasis on "solving the problems," however, opened his strategy right before me. He later acknowledged that what he had learned in the past was in keeping with the best he knew how to do at the time, and that anything he did in the present most likely would be a continuation of his past behavior, yielding the usual temporary results. What he was actually looking for was an outcome which would maintain his relationship with his wife who was tired of his patterns of appeasement. What he needed was to explore an implementation of additional strategies in his behavior that would produce the satisfactory condition in his married life.

He then listed what would be for him a satisfactory condition of marriage, attempting to keep in mind his interpretation of his wife's needs. It was here that I stopped our session because I felt that he had enough raw material to move into a clearer experience of himself and his relationship with his wife. At no point did I solve his "problem" or impose upon him my presuppositions about a specific solution to his pathology. Any of that type of imposition would have been a demonstration of my ability to observe specifically what I know how to observe. In doing that, I would have heard only myself in his words. I would be producing in him a copy of me, because I only know what I currently know how to know, and therefore I could at best superimpose the limits of my knowledge on him. My intuition and/or observations may actually be accurate, but he would still be imprisoned inside the limits of my perception.

By working to solve disease, I am predicated out of discord so that the compositions that are inspired from me, and the ear that I develop are all conditioned by the context out of which my creative venture was birthed—discord. As I argue for my premise, I am limited by my premise because my premise creates me.

As elm trees create elm trees, elm leaves, elm seeds, and elm bark, the "elmness" that is all pervasive within them (although bark, leaf, and seed all look different), does not allow space to explore maple, birch, and especially robin. Limiting the outcome of the encounter because the therapist has a particular 'condition of satisfaction' may not be inclusive enough for the client's current exploration.

Let us take the case of Newtonian physics. The laws of mechanics were a major breakthrough in the scientific development of their time. These laws still hold true today, but what has developed is a technology that transcends the scope of the mechanical paradigm. Thinking had to make the leap to a meta model that included Newtonian physics as a special case in a larger picture.

Let us reevaluate the way we presently frame our therapeutic goals and step outside of our present psychological organization. Let us reformulate our view while maintaining our current knowledge as a special case in the new paradigm.

As modern therapies mature, they are beginning to resemble parts of the ancient approaches to mature psychophysiological maturation. We have need of another dimension to therapy—the holistic approach. This approach emphasizes the treatment of the entire person who may, at any given time, need one or any combination of the above therapeutic approaches. These therapies are spokes in the wheel of human development and all of the spokes must fit the wheel for the wheel to turn.

2
What Is
Yoga?

Yoga comes from the Sanskrit verb root *yuj* which means "to join or unite." The classical approach to yoga is a holistic one that addresses itself to the pursuit of being wholly human. It has been found that a harmonious interaction among the physical, mental, emotional, value, and spiritual dimensions creates a circumstance whereby the genius inherent within the human being naturally awakens.

For centuries yogic sages have applied a vast number of approaches to uncover the natural genius of the human being. Their intent was to tap the innate power of humanness and give it direction through intelligent and spiritual purpose. These approaches have held their relevance across cultures and through times.

In addition to developing dimensions of universality within their techniques, the yogic sages applied themselves in full knowledge that they would be working with different classes of human temperament. As a result they designed a variety of approaches. They realized that the aspirants, upon making a commitment to transformation, would have to face the arduous and sometimes frightening task of discovering how they had become who they were, and after that realization, make the leap into the unknown of what they might become. Not many are competent to make this exploration, let alone take the leap. This subtlety is depicted in the following story.

Long ago in a kingdom in China there was a dragon who terrorized the countryside destroying the farmlands, killing the cattle, and stealing the treasure from the king's vaults. Many great warriors came to slay the dragon. From far across the land, resplendent in battle dress, they rode up the mountain to the dragon's lair never to be seen again. The dragon's reputation became known far and wide until at last not one warrior would step forward to take up the challenge. The country suffered such severe loss that the desperate king offered half of his kingdom to anyone who would kill the dragon.

One courageous knight finally applied for the task and duly set out to engage the dragon in combat. They met and clashed at the base of the mountain in a fierce fight. For three days and three nights they struggled.

The advantage was traded off in a brilliant see-saw contest as they battled ever higher up the hill. At last the warrior backed the dragon into his cave, and with the last thrust of his ebbing strength, delivered the fatal blow. The dragon heaved an agonizing sigh as his body crumbled to the floor of the cave.

Satisfied that the dragon was dead, the knight surveyed the contents of the cave. To his amazement he found it filled with treasures beyond his wildest imaginings. Chests of pure silver stood open, their contents of diamonds, rubies, and pearls spilling to the floor; grains of corn and oats and wheat were heaped in great piles upon golden platters; fruits of every kind formed bright pyramids of colored sweetness. Fine-robed servants stood ready to do his bidding. The very walls were covered with burnished gold, polished to a mirror shine.

The knight was overjoyed at his good fortune and sat down to ponder the future of wealth and ease that would be his. Then out of the corner of his eye he saw, reflecting back at him from the brilliance of the wall, his own image. In astonishment he swung around to face his reflection: he was turning into the dragon!

At that moment he understood what had happened to all the warriors before him. They had been successful. Each of them had in turn slain the dragon, but then, enamored of the treasures in the cave, had become what they had slain—the guardian of the treasure.

The knight turned and ran from the cave as fast as he could run.

It was in this light that the yogic sages sought to generate a quality of genius in their students so that they could attain the insight that they had become the dragon many times. The students had to realize that who they were was a result of the treasures passed down by all who went before. They were conditioned by their species, gender, their position in family and society, their religion, and nationality. All this shaped their encounter with life, and thus the dragon that they were to become.

As we proceed, let us look again at the word yoga and its design. Yoga as a word stands for the process that unfolds from being. The science of yoga is the study and mastery of that process. It is a mistake to confuse yoga with a particular culture because you may alienate yourself from a valuable insight due to the Sanskrit word.

The science of yoga was designed to illuminate first of all the fact that there is a process of becoming the dragon, and then to point out how the unconscious patterns of species, culture, and so forth play the dominant role in creating the human personality. It is through this awareness, followed by the assumption of responsibility for these patterns, that the individual is thus empowered for transformation. Lastly, one's sharpened insight, coupled with the vision and techniques of yogic wisdom, is applied to fathom the possibility of transcending the cave of the mind.

The subjective state of yogi (a practitioner of yoga) would be experienced as a state of being—like male or female. When one awakes in the morning, there is no subjective question of "becoming" male or female; there is only the existential experience of "what is." Yoga is the process of becoming; what one becomes is a consequence of this process.

We will be talking *about* yoga, however, and thus
we will be viewing yoga from an objective perspective.
From this perspective yoga is the study of the mind
and beyond. In the analysis of the mind, yoga studies
the abilities the mind has to make distinctions and to
modify itself in becoming those distinctions. It is
through an understanding of the mind's nature as a
discriminating instrument that we can learn to turn the
mind back towards its source and use it to understand
the essential nature of being. Let us now take a look at
the mind.

The power of being is invested in the mind. In
hindsight, this competency is experienced as expression.
The hindsight is the mind's ability to accept an impression, retain it, and later recall it. This is called memory.
Through the combination of expressing and memory of
the expression, the frame to develop the experience of
an expresser, a personal "I," comes into existence.

The mind has the ability to become anything it
encounters. Within that ability, the humanness of
mind frames awareness out of which can develop a
personal framing or interpretation. It is from here that
we unfold the initial targeting of personal transformation in the yoga science.

Let us say that the "I" is attracted to the science
of biology. "I" then performs the actions that it
interprets will demonstrate the best route to its attraction. "I" may go to study the science of biology with a
reputed master. "I" may read books that are relevant to
biology. "I" may attempt to find employment in the
field. "I" may associate with biologists to discuss and
debate points. All of this will be a means to assimilate,
and be assimilated by, that through which the "I"

is attracted.

Eventually there is a union between the subject "I" and the apparent object "biology" to the point where one no longer makes a distinction between the subject and the object, but refers to the "I" now as "biologist." The two have become one. Grammatically this idea would look like this:

I AM BIOLOGIST

The systematic application of the techniques developed by the yogic sages is directed specifically at unravelling the predicate, the "is-ness," of one's being. For it is by understanding the nature of the "I," that is, the dynamic by which the "I" manifests its creativity and its genius, that the "I" is experienced. Upon expressing ourselves through whichever medium we encounter and choose, our identification with that vehicle becomes so thorough that we are then associated with the object, and in most cases lose ourselves during the assimilation.

"I" can identify itself with any number of objects. The "I," however, becomes so thoroughly involved at particular times with any one of these that it considers itself that object alone. For example, out of the many objects that "I" can become, let us select "mother." "I" now becomes identified with mother:

I AM MOTHER

Next, let's say we have MOTHER, who is angry. Identification has now shifted to ANGRY, and in the identification with anger, access is now not available

to be mother (or biologist, or niece, or daughter)
because "I" is "being," or belonging to, angry.

I AM	BIOLOGIST SISTER MOTHER DAUGHTER NIECE	WHO IS	OBEDIENT LOVING GUILTY ANGRY DEPRESSED

As a result of losing herself in "becoming" angry,
let us further say that the mother later "becomes"
depressed because of her display, and in her depression
"becomes" guilty. So we now have a diagram that
looks like this:

I AM MOTHER WHO IS ANGRY WHO IS DEPRESSED WHO IS GUILTY

The identification has eventually become associated
away from her selfhood and into guilty. The sense of
selfhood is now associated with guilt—quite a psychological distance away from the "I." Her selfhood has
become so thoroughly identified with guilt that were
she to sign a check, she should sign it "guilty."

The first phase of yoga is the technique of discovering the means through which I become what I
think I am. Yoga then takes the subject back to its
source. The rightness or wrongness of any of these
becomings is a value judgment and is basically irrele-
vant in view of discovering the process. What is
important is to discover the source of our being. To
explore whether it is right or wrong to be any of those
things is another experience that "I" manifests and can
become. Among other things "I" can be, being right

22 WHAT IS YOGA?

or wrong are two of them.

In the case of "I" being biologist, mother, daughter, angry, guilty, and so forth, the yogis would have said that the beingness that infuses the I is changeless. But "I" in its expressing becomes biologist at the lab, mother at home with the child, daughter with its parents, sister with its siblings, and so forth. The interpretation through which it expresses itself is its beingness as manifested through its roles. At no time is it changed; it is the same self expressing through the vehicle of science, motherhood, marriage, birth. The knowledge gained from the discovery of the power of "becoming" is then turned towards the subject "I" and the genius of becoming is shone inward to explore and question.

Ultimately the techniques of yoga are designed to cause the mind to disidentify and transcend, but not to disassociate with any specific form. At this stage the mind is in a state of preparedness—a preparedness to become absorbed by anything the first moment it appears. It is unoccupied except with the intent of becoming occupied.

I recall a time when my *gurudev* gathered a small group of us to guide through an intense ten-day period of silence. After supper one day, about the sixth day of silence, I was lying on the diving board above the pond on the grounds of the Himalayan Institute. The water was glassy still. I was lying face down, looking at the water. A lone white cloud stood against the light blue sky. I was observing this in the reflection of the water. Suddenly a bird flew across the sky which shown in reflection below me. I realized that below and above had become one and the same. Extending my gaze to the edge of the pond, I saw the reflection of the violet, yellow and green vegetation growing at the water's edge—a scene at once pointing upward and downward. What was above was below and what was below was above. I marvelled at the mirror images that ringed the pool.

The 180° of upward and downward light created a 360° equation in my mind. The light of the sun reflected off the vegetation into my eyes, and the light of the sun reflected off the vegetation reflecting into the pool and reflected into my eyes. One went upward into the sun behind me and one went upward into the sun in front of me.

There were no words in my thoughts. I lie there unaware of the measurement of time. Yet there was a yearning within me. Without thinking in words, yet knowing clearly, I felt a tug and wondered if I would be able to achieve a state beyond this yearning, for indeed I was wordless. Moving only my eyes, I glanced down the path next to the pool and then scanned the water, listening to the occasional plop of a fish diving into the air and floating back. Suddenly, understanding flowed through my mind. I was waiting to become the next event that came by! The reflection and the sky and I had become one so that there was nothing, because there was only us as I. My mind, in the state of equilibrium, was waiting with full intent to become the next thing that came up—be it a fish jumping, a bird flying across one of the skies, or a person to observe as he walked down the path.

The dynamic technique of yoga science is to skillfully, purposefully, take the mind to a state where it is not involved in being anything in particular. It is in that state that one can then turn inward to explore. When the mind is not in that state, it is constantly involved with, ultimately enmeshed in, and assimilated by those classes of perceptions.

The achievement of insight into the process of becoming is critical in the development of the yogic mentality. Yogic sages do not consider choicelessness to be dysfunctional behavior. They have devised and systematized processes for achieving this goal. These techniques are relevant to human growth regardless if one's intention is enlightenment or improving the quality of his life.

It is this body of knowledge that I offer to the therapeutic paradigm, for I have found that the goals of yoga and the goals of modern therapy do contain areas of relatedness. My purpose is to implement yoga therapy as an adjunct to the already existing therapeutic programs. In the case of each program my intention is for the utilization of yoga science to expand the arena in which therapist and client may relate. In this way both gain a deeper awareness, together with a wider range of skills, to creatively explore the mind.

The great teachers of life who used the yoga systems understood that in order to employ transformation through the holistic model, they had to relate through the differences of the people who came to study with them. It is because of these differences that various systems of yoga were developed.

There are many types of yoga, some of which are peculiar to specific traditions. There are, however, nine classical approaches. These are: union through devotion *(bhakti yoga)*, action *(karma yoga)*, intellect *(jnana yoga)*, meditation *(raja yoga)*, control of the life force *(hatha yoga)*, awakening of the unconscious *(kundalini yoga)*, the power of word *(mantra yoga)*, the power of sound *(nada yoga)*, and the absorption of levels of consciousness *(laya yoga)*.

For the purposes of our discussion we will limit our remarks to the first six listed. Although there are many applications of these types of yoga, we will confine our discussion to those aspects that are complimentary to the therapy model.

The first three yogas—devotion, action, and intellect—are called the yogas of life. They are said to be so because in the process of living, the involvement with life naturally incorporates these three approaches.

The Yoga of Devotion
Bhakti Yoga

Devotion is the investment of emotional intensity in the areas in which one chooses to be committed. In life, the power to move arises when we make a commitment. Commitment is the quality through which we make our word real. When we commit, we decide to invent or become our decision by investing our life force in bringing our decision into reality.

The relevance this has for therapy is exemplified in many ways, two of which follow. First, we become involved with whatever aspect of life we engage because of our attraction to it. If there is no attraction, there is no involvement. It is this attraction that gives direction to our creativity. Second is commitment. We make commitments based on our attractions, and it is out of commitment that our attraction takes on form. It is a power of our being. It is what moves us. Commitment is the love that the lover expresses toward the beloved, be it mundane or divine. *Bhakti* is surrender in order to be filled with the object of surrender.

The Yoga of Action
Karma Yoga

The yoga of action, at its first stage, is to act skill-fully. Another way to say that is, find out how things work and get on the good side of them. It is important to be clear about accepting "how it is." Some of us don't like the way it is, and as a result constantly suffer the blows of being trapped in our interpretation of reality. This concept is very clearly explained in the nursery rhyme:

> Row, row, row your boat
> Gently down the stream.
> Merrily, merrily, merrily, merrily
> Life is but a dream.

The state of rowing your boat down the stream is the enlightened state, because the way things go is the way they are going. You can choose to attempt to go against the nature of life as it is experienced in the human context. However, at some point you must surrender to the existential reality, and it is from there that the doors to the practical (and later a transcendent) experience of reality can be open.

The Yoga of Intellect
Jnana Yoga

The yoga of intellect is a systematic process whereby the student goes from the unreal to the real, from a single view and unexamined experience toward the willingness and ability to really experience "what is." The thought process is an important ingredient in this type of yoga, for the student utilizes intelligent exploration via contemplation in the context of a commitment to real-izing what is.

Let us use as an example a yogic seeker sitting on the bank of a stream. In looking at the stream, he muses that the stream, the earth, the vegetation are in reality all one as material substance. This helps him to realize that his body, too, shares with them in being part and parcel of the same material reality. Pursuing further, he realizes that his mind, though subtler, is the same reality at a more refined level. And logically deducing that the thoughts which he thinks, being a product of the mind, are none other than that same reality, he then intellectually realizes through his systematic probing that everything is indeed all one.

The value of this approach is made real through his commitment to explore truth, for it is from there that he is willing to entertain the idea that his existence as an ego may not be separate from that of water, the planet, or whatever else he might have the ability to experience.

Any of these three yogas may be given to a seeker as the path that best suits him in his real-izing of "what is." The next three paths of yoga are said not to be apparently inherent in life. Again, they are paths suited to particular types of personalities.

The Yoga of Meditation
Raja Yoga

The yoga of meditation is designed to unravel the neuroses created by oneself in life. When one meditates the obstacles that one creates for oneself become glaringly evident. I would like to correct a common misconception about meditation. In the beginning meditation does appear to smooth out and ease one's life, but quite readily afterwards one's limits are encountered. Life seems to speed up, giving one an opportunity to clarify what he is doing in life by bringing up his foibles, biases and stupidity. When this happens often enough in a short period of time, one can acknowledge these limits for what they are and transform oneself if one has the courage to do so.

When one sits quietly and meditates, one is sitting in the middle of the memories of the mind. One is living very specifically with who he has become. There is absolutely no notion of escape in meditation. Some may attempt to use it as such, but with proper guidance that is easily corrected.

The Yoga of Control of Vital Forces
Hatha Yoga

The yoga of controlling the vital forces has been popularly known as the physical side of yoga. Some people mistakenly identify the whole of this science with physical postures. Postures are only one avenue of hatha yoga, and there are only a few yogis who focus exclusively on this aspect. I would like to utilize the Sanskrit term for this yoga because the sound itself has to do with what it is. *Hatha* is a symbolic word. *Ha* means "sun" and *tha* means "moon." Hatha yoga, then, is a re-presentation of the union between opposites. Hatha is a harmonization of left brain and right brain activities through the energy system of the body gained specifically through control of the glands, nervous system and breath. It is through the control of these unconscious functions that the powers of the physical human being are put at the service of the aspirant. We will point out later, in the chapter on yoga postures, the psychological significance of the postures and the impact that they make upon conscious and unconscious development, maintenance and transformation.

The Yoga of Awakening the Unconscious
Kundalini Yoga

The sages knew, through their own experience, that in order to unravel the brilliant warp and woof of human reality, the full potential and genius of the mind must be at hand. The greatest portion of the mind's potential, however, is held out of awareness; only a small part of the mind is consciously employed.

In our desire to be safe we have imprisoned our genius in the bottle of our defenses. In order to exist as a full human being we must release our genie—the guardian spirit of our wisdom, creativity and power. Then as responsible partners all parts of our being can apply themselves to the subtle dimensions of existence.

In order for things to change, we have to change. Space for transformation to appear must be invented. So any change that takes place is the willingness to invent a space where transformation can emerge. This is the goal of the masters. They may indeed have an idea about the direction they would like the aspirant to take, but rather than attempt to force him into a mold, they create the circumstances by which reality can be known.

By studying the various dimensions we human beings must pass through in self-realization, the sages devised processes that would make the dynamic of mind visible. These processes serve as ingredients in the mortar that holds together life's experiences in such a way that these experiences become the foundation for transformation.

3
The
Addiction
Process

It is inconclusively known what causes one individual, and not another, to be abusive and addicted to substances. Investigation into genetics, body chemistry, psychological dysfunction, family history, and hypoglycemia, to name a few causes, are currently being conducted to ascertain what are the predispositions to chronic abusive-addictive behavior. In exploring the dependency process and describing a typical treatment program, I will be specifying alcohol abuse in my metaphors since it is the most abused substance in the West today.

Below I will categorize some types of substances and abuses that are typical. In the rest of the chapter, however, alcohol will be utilized as a symbol to represent the syndrome of all of these addicting substances. The syndrome of alcohol abuse is sufficiently similar to other substance abuses that the juxtaposition will hold up adequately.

The first group of drugs is considered to be addicting regardless of the user or his chemistry. Class A drugs, such as heroin, morphine, and opium, fall into this category. Their effect on the human organism is very severe, and the physical and emotional dysfunction comes much earlier in the cycle of addiction than with other substances.

A second group of substances commonly abused is alcohol, marijuana, cocaine, amphetamines, tranquillizers, and the like. We do have an arena of usage of some of these mood-altering substances that by and large is considered to be socially acceptable. This is the domain called responsible usage. Some of these drugs are prescribed, but harmful dependency can still evolve from them. Such is the case of valium.

In a situation where pressures are intense, the strategy for treatment by many attending physicians is often to write a prescription for a tranquillizer or an amphetamine, depending upon the desired direction of the mood to be altered. In my view this is not serving the patient in most cases. What takes place is that the chemical causes the emotional pressure to be put temporarily out of awareness—on the back burner, so to speak. When the chemical wears off, the emotional issues come back to the fore. This will then require repeated involvement with the chemical.

Over a period of time the emotional issues stack up outside of awareness, and the enormity of this emotional heap becomes too great to deal with. Then, just in order to get through the day, medication becomes essential. This instance applies to all the substances in this group, whether they are prescribed, or elicited across the counter or on the street.

Hallucinogenics constitute the third group of mood-altering chemicals. These include LSD, peyote, and other hallucinogenic plants. Historically, these substances were often used by cultures for ecstatic experiences associated with religious ritual. In our culture we have taken them to the point where there are harmful consequences to the brain. The abuse of hallucinogenics can result in the damage of brain cells causing the brain to lose its capacity for clarity. It takes extensive abuse before this begins to be evident, but even serial usage can fuzz thinking and productivity.

The fourth category of chemical substances includes refined sugar, caffeine, nicotine, and in some cases, salt. Much research has been done on the effects of refined sugar on the sugar-sensitive individual. Its effect on blood sugar immediately and dramatically changes the climate of the brain and causes severe emotional dysfunction in these individuals. Researchers are finding that many people in institutions for emotional disorders are actually sugar sensitive (see chapter on Diet, p. 107).

Along these lines is the puzzle of food alergy. Some people experience extreme mood shifts, such as tremendous anger, in response to certain kinds of nourishment. This is similar to the response to sugar of sugar-sensitive people. It is apparent that salt has the same emotional effect on some people, while others react violently after ingesting eggs, milk, or wheat.

The harmful consequences associated with nicotine reside very strongly in the direct effect of this drug on the body. As we shall see below in our story about harmful dependency, a person's relationship with his chemical becomes the most important relationship in his life. Smoking is a classic example of the primary love relationship with a chemical. Cigarette smoking impacts other people as much as it impacts the smoker, yet the smoker feels defiant against those who request that he alter his behavior. With the wealth of scientific evidence so prevalent about the dangers of nicotine, it is dumbfounding to see parents smoking in a car filled with their children, in full knowledge of the effect that their smoking has upon the children's health.

I would like to point out here a mentality that permeates our North American lifestyle. In a large sense we choose not to be responsible for our own psychological and physical maintenance. In this lies the core of our abusive conduct. As we seek emotional relief through alcohol, marijuana and tranquillizers, we seek physical relief from the pain of our overindulgence in food through digestive aids. Rather than eating responsibly, we abuse our bodies and then introduce an external agent to take care of us. We follow this same pattern associated with symptoms that the body produces to notify us of dysfunction. We will anesthetize ourself with an analgesic rather than investigate the source of our pain. It is like knocking out the red oil light on the dashboard of our car, thinking that we have solved the problem of low oil.

The last category of addiction is associated with anorexia and bulimia. The prevalence of these two diseases seems to be a modern phenomenon. It appears to plague women much more than men, though both can exhibit this abberent pattern of physical and emotional addiction. The impact of anorexia (starving the body of food) and bulimia (gorging with food and then regurgitating it) is significant in terms of their interference with body physiology. Because it does not provide essential nourishment for the brain and other organs necessary to maintain the organism, these addictive behaviors are critical. As we have seen, and will see further in the chapter on diet, once the brain is starved, the quality of thinking begins to deteriorate, increasing the predisposition toward dysfunctional thinking and emotional upset.

Theories of Addiction and Treatment

There are a number of theories about how the relationship between the addictive substance and the abusive-addictive person is initiated and maintained. Some of these are: incompatible body chemistry with the substance, family history, inherent weakness in the soul's ability to withstand temptation, and psychological disorder.

Many philosophies, each with its own individual theory of treatment, have been developed and implemented as treatment models. We here list the major ones.

1.   One theory is responsible usage. This theory proposes that the dependent person can responsibly use the chemical again at some point in his life.

2.   The theory of substitutive drugs is based on the

use of another substance to take the place of previously addictive substances. This is exemplified in the methodone program in which methodone is substituted for heroin.

3. Next is the theory of alternative high. Here, there is an attempt to substitute a natural means of getting "high" (euphoria) so that the client will switch from the relationship of using harmful substances. Mountain climbing, wilderness survival, and breathing practices are some of the activities substituted as alternatives to the drug.

4. Another theory is that of seeking intercession from a power greater than oneself in prayer.

5. In the support group theory, the experience of others and the support to remain chemically free is lent to the recovering person by those who have already achieved recovery. In addition, a forum for getting unresolved emotional turmoil out into the open is provided.

6. The next theory is the well-known Twelve Steps of Alcoholics Anonymous (AA). They include affirmations, prayer, support groups, and confession.

7. A relatively new theory employs the use of amino acids, vitamin supplements, and sound nutrition while investigating the client's inclinations toward sugar-sensitivity. The program is augmented with therapeutic counseling.

8. In the rest of this chapter I will be speaking specifically about a theory of abuse and treatment called the disease model. Though not totally at one with all the other above theories, the disease model generalizes sufficiently in my view to broadly delineate the addictive process for our purposes.

It is the view of the disease model that involvement with a chemical is learned. Once the process of involvement is learned, the results of the learned behavior are specifically sought after by the personality. Involvement is generated by learning what is called the mood swing.

When a person becomes involved with a chemical (in this case àlcohol), he moves from his typical homeostatic state toward a state of perceived euphoria. He then returns to his normal state of homeostasis. This swing towards euphoria and return to normal is called the mood swing.

This learning and eventual seeking is not limited to the abusive-addictive personality, but is shared by the human population at large. The difference is how far one goes in seeking euphoria and the price one is willing to pay to achieve and maintain it.

In seeking the mood swing through alcohol, an individual finds that one drink is good and two drinks are better. He finds this formula works every time. This is the learning process. There is a continual movement towards a perceived euphoria as seen in the following chart.*

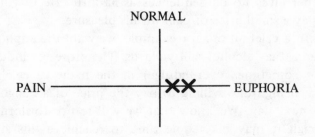

* The Feeling Charts were designed by Vernon E. Johnson of the Johnson Institute of Minneapolis, Minnesota, and are used with his permission.

At this point of involvement with learning the mood swing, one returns to normal quite easily without much physical or emotional cost. The first stage of learning has taken place. In the next stage, one drinks even more, and he finds that more can be better still. Again the results can be counted upon. There is always a return to normal, but as one consumes more, there is a minor rebound into an area of pain to the point where physical discomfort can be experienced the next day.

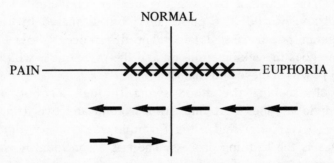

This is the stage in which the average consumer of mood-altering substances finds himself. In this pattern he perceives no consequences as harmful. He is willing to pay a small price of pain for his pleasure.

In a celebration, for example, we want the euphoric release that alcohol will yield us. Therefore we indulge (and sometimes over-indulge) in the name of celebration, being quite willing to pay the price of a hangover the next day. We know that we will return to normal, though it may take some time to reachieve this state of ease. Social drinkers sometimes find themselves in this position and for most of them the occasional overindulgence is not a problem.

There is a point, however, where some individuals in seeking the mood swing move into the area of pain in the process of their usage. An expanded definition of pain becomes necessary at this stage. As the quantity of alcohol consumed is increased, information from the cerebral cortex is inhibited, blocking values and short-term memory. As a result behavior is generated that would not be exhibited under ordinary circumstances and/or remorse. Now a psychological pain accompanies the physical discomfort of a hangover.

To illustrate, let us follow John into harmful dependency.

At a gathering, John drinks and becomes the life of the party. His behavior, however, starts to get out of hand. He becomes inappropriate with other guests and generally acts in a way that is incongruent in his cultural setting, embarrassing to his wife, and at odds with his own values in his normal state. This embarrassment and contradiction move him into the area of pain while seeking the mood swing.

When John wakes up the next morning, he requires longer than usual to return to normal, due to his physical discomfort, the mood of his wife, and his own remorse over his behavior of the night before. He must make peace with his body, he must make peace with his wife, and he must assuage the guilt of his inappropriate behavior before his peers. Although the price has become higher, he still eventually returns to normal.

It is somewhere in here that the fuzzy line of addictive behavior can be recognized. Some individuals explore this area but do not experience addiction;

John, however, finds himself in this same predicament again and again, regardless of his remorse and his resolve not to repeat it. It frightens him to acknowledge that he is out of control. Let us follow his experience further:

John is again at an office celebration at the president's home. He has promised his wife and himself that he will behave more appropriately this time. He arrives at the party, heads straight for the bar, and begins to drink in order to come down from work and get in the mood for the party. It is not long before he finds himself in the same predicament as before. He is flirting with Martha, the president's wife, dancing on the table, and talking at the top of his voice. He remembers his resolve with himself to respect the norms of social behavior. He remembers his promises to his wife. Yet here he is again, as if he were out of control and had no choice. His values, his integrity, his love for his spouse, friends, and career have apparently been set aside.

The next morning John awakens alone in bed and remembers that he has done it again. He rolls out of bed with a tremendous headache. He looks at himself in the mirror, bedraggled, red-eyed, and wearing the remnants of the night before and the morning after. He remembers now all the drinks that he had when he first arrived at the party and thinks to himself, "That Martha! If it weren't for her I wouldn't have drunk so much before supper. She was late with dinner, so what could I do but drink on an empty stomach? Obviously it is her fault that I got drunk. Anyway, it was a dull party, and all I did was liven it up. If it weren't for me, the whole damn party would have been a flop."

He showers and shaves, and while dressing thinks about the party again. Now he remembers flirting with Martha. He thinks to himself, "Ah, she's been coming on to me for months now. I don't know why Phyllis [his wife] is blaming me. It's not my fault that the woman is crazy about me."

He sits down to tie his shoes and remembers how everyone laughed when he was trying to climb up on the diving board. He totally forgets the panic of the group as he fell in the pool, not knowing how to swim.

He walks down the stairs, whistling, adjusting his tie, and enters the kitchen with a smile on his face. He ignores the tear-streaked face of his angered wife and says, "Good morning!" She glares at him, and in her anger remonstrates with him about his broken promises, obnoxious behavior, and apparent non-concern for her feelings. He angrily retorts that he doesn't know why she is making such a big deal about nothing. All he did was have a few drinks and a little fun. She is just jealous of his ability to get along with people so well, and rather than spend time with a shrew, he will go out and have breakfast by himself until she can be more civil.

John has just utilized a strategy called sincere delusion. Because his behavior has been so inappropriate according to his own value system, because he promised his wife and himself that he would not do it again, and because he is frightened he has done it, John has built a wall of defenses around himself. He employs selective recollection of memories so he can interpret the events of his life in a certain way. He must maintain an image of himself that he can live with, which also allows him to continue his use of alcohol.

In the addiction process, first the person takes the chemical, then the chemical takes the person, and in the last stage, the chemical takes the chemical, for there is no longer any person left. The relationship to the chemical becomes the most important relationship to the person. Family, job, and values are secondary.

In the case of John, we find that he sincerely believes his defenses because he needs to. Compounding the tragedy of his own mind is the fact that after repeated occurrences of self-deception, lies, and broken promises, his wife and children begin to doubt their own sanity. John so thoroughly believes his deluded reality that he causes them to question their own. In addition, they begin to adjust their reality to fit his, and become as much a victim of his dependency as he is. Remember, John has woven a skillful and intricate cage around himself to protect his very narrow piece of well-being. He can present such a good argument that those close to him are sometimes duped by his logic. They begin to believe that people really are against Dad or don't really understand her husband.

This is why chemical dependency therapy views chemical dependency as a family illness, whereby the entire family must be involved in the therapeutic process.

The next step in the addiction process occurs when John, in seeking the mood swing, goes so deeply into the area of pain that in order to return to normal he must drink. This is called drinking to be normal. John is now living constantly in an area of pain. If he stops usage of the chemical, he will slide back into the area of pain—the psychological pain of guilt imposed by his values over his inappropriate behavior, and the recognition of disapproval from his loved ones. In weaving his protective screen to keep out pain, he does not realize that it will crystallize, trapping him inside. He needs to not experience—to not see, hear, or feel the reality of his predicament. It is essential for him to block off the memory of behavior that is in conflict with his values in order to maintain a self-image that supports a sense of security and painlessness in his life. He needs to ignore the harmful consequences threatening his sense of well-being. The pain inflicted upon his loved ones and himself stands around him like a spectre, casting a shadow of guilt and low self-esteem, and making him feel powerless to do it any other way. To illustrate, let us continue John's addiction process.

Incidents like the party begin to be the norm for John. He values his relationship with the chemical more and more. In addition to his drinks to unwind at the end of the work day, he begins to drink at the lunch hour, coming back to the office later and later. He even occasionally has a drink early in the morning. He justifies this behavior as necessary to take the edge off, complaining that if upper management and those below him would become more organized, his job wouldn't be so stressful. "If those guys at the top didn't have it so easy, and would just get off their duffs, my job wouldn't be so hard. Besides, the shipping department thinks of no one but themselves and can't seem to get anything out on time. A guy's got to drink just to do a good job around here."

On his way home to attend his daughter's dance recital, John stops for a couple of quick ones and doesn't arrive home until 9 P.M., missing the recital and leaving his daughter to feel that he doesn't care about her. He continues to create more and more pain as a result of his relationship with the chemical. He loves his chemical more than he loves himself, his family, his career. His behavior (which is really chemical behavior), demonstrates it. There is more and more that his self-image cannot tolerate or acknowledge about himself. He cannot hide, so he enters the last stage of drinking. He now drinks in order to feel normal, seeking the alcohol lift to rescue him from the pain that hounds his heels like a fury.

He tries to handle this problem alone, failing many times. He is "stacking up" a pile of pain that is insurmountable. The alcohol has allowed him to temporarily put aside pain, which in turn creates more pain. The accrued emotional debt becomes too great to handle, burying him under a mountain that crushes him with its weight. Reality now becomes a narrow corridor. He is walled in by the defenses that keep him safe from the dangerous terrain of the strewn casualties behind him.

Corrective Processes Associated with Chemical Dependency Therapies

There are two important steps involved in the initiation of therapeutic intervention and treatment.

The first step in the corrective process is to get the client to acknowledge that he has a problem with a drug. As is typical of the human condition, when one is enmeshed in a strategy, one is usually the last to see his "stuckness." Typically a crisis, the courts, or a well-orchestrated confrontation with professional assistance are the common occurrences that bring the severity of the problem to light.

For example, John's physician may inform him that his liver is malfunctioning and that premature death is his eventual route. Or John may run afoul of the law in an alcohol-related incident causing a perceptive judge to dictate that he be evaluated to ascertain whether or not he is chemically dependent. Or John's family and friends, out of their concern for him, may seek professional assistance to confront his behavior.

Let us continue our scenario with John's family, friends, and employer confronting him. Out of their love for him they sought a skilled professional who assisted them in confronting John's destructive behavior. His wife had attempted to confront him before by herself, but it ended up in a name-calling shoutdown, each of them becoming over-emotional. It ended with her walking away, thinking that perhaps she needed psychological care and John had been right all along.

This time the therapist kept John from dividing and conquering, which was a skill that he had ably developed. Each member was instructed to carefully write out an abberent event with John listing dates, times, and circumstances so that they could read the event to him and show how they were personally affected by his behavior. By reading their reports, they avoided being clouded with emotion at the confrontation, or not being able to recall what they were going to say due to anger or threats from John.

A meeting was arranged at which John was tricked

into attending. (He would not attend a meeting of his own free will to meet his pain.) When John arrived everyone was waiting to confront him with the effect he was having on their lives. John felt set up and betrayed. This did not fit his narrow view of reality. His response at being thwarted was to become enraged. After two hours of irrefutable evidence, however, he finally began to see through his defenses to what was taking place.

One instance was related by John's daughter, Peggy, who, through tears, told her father why she never brought her friends home. Once he had been lying passed out on the sofa when she walked through the living room with a group of her friends. Then in a drunken stupor, he made a pass at one of the girls. His daughter informed him of how embarrassed she was, and that she was now afraid to ever bring anyone home again. The last thing that John wanted to do was to hurt his daughter.

With all the evidence from each member stacked before him, John agreed that he had a problem. He would go into treatment for help. At the same time, the family was brought into the therapy process because over the years it had learned to tolerate his abusive-addictive behavior purely as a result of living with him. The family unconsciously supported him in his behavior by establishing a relationship with his chemical and then relating to it because John was not there to contact.

The second step in the corrective process is the necessity of taking the client off of the chemicals. As long as the individual is still using a drug, the therapy cannot effectively be applied to the person. It will be applied to the chemical. This is why some therapeutic encounters are not successful. The client is not identified as being chemically dependent, and as a result, the therapist does not meet with any degree of success because he does not have a person in the room, but a chemical.

Let us take a last look at John. In the protected environment of the therapeutic community, John can take the risk of existing without his defenses. "Feelings are facts" is one of the hallmarks of the disease model. In the past it was important for John to stay out of contact with his feelings because his pain was stored there. Now he is encouraged quite strongly to acknowledge the validity of his feelings.

Upon release from therapy, John is encouraged, or even required, to continue with support groups, because the desire to reestablish the relationship with a drug will persist. Having someone in the same boat, so to speak, is of great value.

4 Addiction: The Yoga Parallel

We have seen in the preceding chapter a description of the process whereby one slowly and unerringly becomes so thoroughly involved with dysfunctional behavior that one's original personality is lost. It is hidden behind the now dominant sets of behaviors imposed by the outside agent of drugs.

The yogic sages have written much about this paradigm of addiction. They refer to it in Sanskrit as the philosophy of the *kleshas*. The model of "becoming" in the second chapter (biologist is mother) is based on the first two steps of this *klesha* philosophy.

The word *klesha* means "source of pain." By this is
meant if one becomes secondarily involved with sets
of behavior that one has generated, one is in a painful
state. This is so because a secondary state of behavior
does not hold the full potency of the first, or primary
state. As a result of this limiting identification, one's
power to produce results will be diminished to what is
available in the secondary state. Thus one loses contact
with the validity and power of his original state.

Basically this covers the gist of the first two *kleshas*
in how one becomes wrongly identified with a secondary element. The next two *kleshas* go on to say that the
secondary state has its own set of preferences, and as
a result of being identified with this state, one becomes
identified with the preferences. The preferences are
generalized into the two following statements:

The attraction that is associated with pleasure

The repulsion that is associated with pain.

Yoga Sutras, II. 7-8

The key words in these two phrases are "attraction"
and "repulsion," for it is not the pleasure nor the pain
that creates difficulty, but the need to attract or maintain the pleasure at all costs, and the need to repulse or
avoid the pain at all costs. Emotions and values are
generated in association with this attraction and repulsion.

The last *klesha* is formed in recognition that once
one has so thoroughly enmeshed himself in the secondary state to the point where the primary state is all but
lost, or at least invisible, the sense of identity or selfhood

has become thoroughly invested in the secondary state. This being so, the drive for self-preservation is connected to preserving the secondary state, the secondary state now being as one's own self. As the *sutra* says,

> The identification is so thorough as to fool
> even the wise.
>
> Yoga Sutras, II.9

This view of becoming is the etiology of addiction. The sages look upon the pain of misidentification as the pain of addiction—the thorough possession by a force that is inconsistent with one's essential nature. Based on the *kleshas* as the addiction process seen from yoga, and positing the addiction process as seen from the disease model, I draw the following parallel:

YOGA MODEL	DISEASE MODEL
1. Self becomes non-self	1. Person takes the chemical
2. Non-self considers itself the self	2. Chemical takes the person
3. Non-self clings to life	3. Chemical takes the chemical

Let us consider how the identification process comes into being in light of addiction from the yogic viewpoint. This process will be depicted in the following play. It is an example of the above-mentioned transference of identity to the secondary state and the eventual exclusive identification of self with the behavior of ego. There is an obvious disregard of the behavior of primary intelligence or genius.

SELF
A Play in One Act

CHARACTERS: REAL SELF, who is the source of existence and illuminates the mind through its innate, primary and transpersonal genius
SELF, who is the conscious part of every mind, and is the child in the play
EGO, which is the unconscious part of every mind, and is the child in diapers in our play.

(Enter stage left a small child, named SELF, and stage right a beautiful, divine spirit, named REAL SELF)

REAL SELF: I am so excited about our partnership and new adventure! I have waited to express myself in this world for a long time. You are the important opportunity for that express-ion. I hope that you will have the same feelings as I do. I have so much to say, and I'm looking forward to enjoying a brief respite of temporary existence through you if you agree.

SELF   (In obvious awe of the splendor of this Being before him) What am I to do?

REAL SELF: First of all, before you can do anything, you must learn to communicate in the world. Here, let me teach you how to move. . . . Good! Now let me teach you a little bit about thinking.

(Enter stage left EGO in diapers)

EGO: Did someone say thinking? That's what I like to do best of all! As a matter of fact, that's all I can do.

(REAL SELF and SELF ignore the monolog of the newcomer).

REAL SELF: Now you need to learn how to walk. Try it.

SELF: (Falling) This is painful. I keep falling down!

EGO: (Following around behind SELF and experiencing all the sensations of SELF)   OUCH!!

REAL SELF: Keep trying. You're doing fine.

SELF: (Looking out at the audience)   But people are laughing at me.

REAL SELF: That's all right. Let's take the risk and learn to walk anyway.

EGO: Is all this really worth it? It's too painful. Let's stop. . . . OUCH!   See there? You fell again.

REAL SELF: Keep going. Good. Now let's tackle speaking.

SELF: But they're laughing again!

EGO: Well, I guess that's all right. At least I'm getting

some attention. You two aren't paying any attention to me!

REAL SELF: Now that you've learned to walk and talk, let's try personal relationships.

EGO: Oh! I'm good at that! I remember everything that I've ever done. Remember, my job is remembering.

SELF (Walking closer to REAL SELF) Mommy said to let Johnny play with my toys. What should I do?

REAL SELF: You've learned how to think. What will you do?

EGO: Remember the last time this happened, kiddo? You got a spanking for being selfish!

SELF: (Disregarding EGO and asserting himself) I do not want to share.

EGO and SELF together: OUCH!!

SELF.   I just got spanked!

REAL SELF: It's still important for you to learn to express yourself freely. Just look at the situation and then decide what to do. That is my teaching to you.

EGO: Forget him! I don't want to get spanked any

more. Let's do what Mommy says.

SELF. (Turning to look at EGO for the first time) Hmmm. . . That sounds like a good idea.

EGO: You should have listened to me before. You should have listened to me yesterday when we ate that cookie. I told you we'd be punished if we told the truth. But NO. You had to listen to REAL SELF! You told the truth and we got punished. He doesn't feel any of the pain! He just wants to take all those risks. (Grumbling, he continues) All he talks about day and night is taking risks. He keeps giving us new ideas to try out and gets us in trouble!

SELF: But he's so smart. He taught me how to walk, and how to talk. Where would you be if he hadn't done that?

EGO: I know. I know. But now we're bigger and he's just getting us in trouble. We don't need him. Won't it be more fun if people liked us and didn't yell at us so much? (Aside to the audience, and motioning with his thumb to REAL SELF) That guy is dangerous! I'd better figure out how to get rid of him.

SELF: Well, not getting in trouble would be safer, and nicer.

REAL SELF: (Silently looks on and listens)

SELF: Here comes Johnny. I bet they're going to make me share my toys again.

EGO: Now look (putting his hand around SELF's shoulder conspiratorially) the last time you tried to assert your independence, we got a spanking. Now, we both know the reason we got spanked was because we made Mom and Dad look bad. This time, let the kid play with your toys. I know that will work.

SELF: Well, all right. Here goes. . . . Hey! You're right. Mom and Dad are so happy with me.

EGO: See, we did it. Stick with me, kid. The next time Johnny comes over, I'm going to let him play with *my* toys again. (He puts his hands behind his back and begins to strut around the stage.)

SELF: (Follows EGO around the stage the way EGO had been following him previously) OK.

EGO: I'm hungry.

SELF: OK.

EGO: And I know what else I'm going to do. I'm going to tell Mommy that I love her.

SELF: OK.

EGO: (Walking toward the wings)   I think I want

a cookie. . . .

SELF: (Following EGO) OK.

EGO: (Offstage) Now, I'm going to take this stupid diaper off. It's embarrassing.

SELF: (Offstage, and in a fading voice) OK. . .

REAL SELF: (Stands stage center alone. Lights fade to dark and REAL SELF stands, shining in the darkness. Forgotten.)

* * *

Although our play ends on the note of self's identification with the behavior of ego, this identification remains only until self and ego mature and, in partnership, seek the Real Self again.

The Five Skandas

The system of the five *skandas* is another conceptual schema that describes the formation of the sense of "I," or the ego, as the origin of human consciousness. They are the five active elements that constitute the human personality in time and space. These aggregates are: material form, sensation, perception, motivation and rational consciousness. On the one hand they prove to be valuable, but on the other hand, they can be imprisoning if selected as one's only criteria, thus forming compulsive behavior.

In the addiction process we saw that when the chemical took the chemical all of the traces of the original person disappeared. The *kleshas* and the *skandas* disclose that if one identifies with the ego, all traces of the original self are eliminated from awareness. The *kleshas* point out human involvement with pain; the *skandas* point out human involvement with ignorance.

In the beginning there was no-thing. The word "nothing" does not necessarily mean that there is or is not an existence; it merely indicates that a sense of separateness or I-ness is not present. For example, the ocean is its ocean self. If, for our analogy's sake, there were only ocean, then there would be no ocean because there would be no thing else to compare it with or identify it as something. In the ocean the potential for drops of water is fully present, but they may or may not appear. There can be millions and billions of drops of water, yet if at no time the drops considered themselves to be other than ocean, then at all times ocean alone exists. Truth is that ocean alone exists. The appearance of I (or separateness) comes into being when one drop considers itself to be other than the ocean. The only alteration is that the ocean as a drop now considers itself to be a drop rather than the ocean. The drop is confusing itself as the source of its own existence.

It is here that I-ness comes into existence, for out of the immensity (the no-thing-ness), a light appears. It is the ego in the void, that which is void of attachment to separateness, crying, "It is I." The I-ness seeks to maintain its self-existence and to do so, must ignore the reality of "there is only one" or "there is truly none." It must maintain its separateness in order to achieve and preserve its sense of identity. It asserts and maintains this by viewing things as other than itself. It creates in its perception a "thou." It becomes important to keep the separateness of I-thou, because as long as it can separate and remain inside of its narrow boundaries, it knows that it exists, and it ignores any data that would contradict that.

You see, it is not necessarily true that there is no multiplicity prior to the mention of the ego. Let us take a forest of trees for an example. All of the trees know that there is a forest, and yet they see and feel themselves individually. They know that they are all forest. At the point where one of these separates in thought from its connectedness to the forest and perceives itself to be other than what is, separateness then comes into multiplicity. So now we have "I," which creates thou. "I" maintains the existence of thou out of a need to continually validate itself as separate. Now that thou, or other, is out there, "I" must explore and examine it to see if the other "I" poses a threat to its existence. When there is two there is fear.

Based on the feedback that "I" gets from its perception of thou, "I" interprets what responses would be appropriate to its continuance. First, does it support the existence or continuance of I? If so, "I" wants to consume or assimilate or draw it near. Second, does it threaten the existence or continuance of "I"? If so, then "I" develops defenses to protect itself. Third, does it remind "I" of the reality of no-thing? If so, "I" ignores it or puts it out of its awareness.

"I" has access to storing information and will pigeonhole all of the data that is pertinent to continue its existence, whether it is assimilating, defending, or ignoring. It labels the pigeonholes for convenient reference with names or conceptual psychological structures, and creates a map of reality out of which is structured conscious perception of that which is other.

This is all done in ignorance of the fact that it has created the entire screen of reality. Emotions and thoughts are then generated and utilized in association with maintaining the reality that has been organized. In view of the reality being organized around defensiveness, the defensive posture tends towards self-preservation rather than towards exploration for "what is." We must remember that the "I" chooses in this case to ignore "what is" because from its perspective, to experience or explore "what is" threatens the validity of its existence.

The Six Strategies

This schema then proposes that there are six strategies, one of which tends to be favored by the "I" to maintain its sense of separateness. Seeing through these strategies assists in the waking up process. All of us will recognize that we indeed use one or more of these strategies. It is important to recognize one's favorite behavior—the one that comes up unconsciously, as if one had no choice.

For example, I, myself, have gotten to the point that whenever I find that I am embroiled in my favorite strategy, I automatically know that I am stuck. I now no longer question it. I assume that I am in there to protect my view and that truth has nothing to do with what I am about. In hindsight I find that I am indeed less than resourceful at these times, and thus automatically suspect my clarity.

The Strategy of Being Right

The first strategy is being right all the time. Some people are always right, always have an answer ready, and employ this strategy to prove that others are wrong. This is the "all together" strategy—an answer for everything.

The shortcoming of the all-together strategy is that "I" is still supporting the duality that there is a right and a wrong. (This is not to say that there is no wrong). The duality of being caught in right and wrong is thinking that right and wrong came out of a different place; they actually have their source in the same context. Their reality is dependent upon each other, and is relative to the perceptual base of the interpreter. To think that the wrong must be eliminated while the right must be encouraged, because the right is supreme, is to be caught in a web of your own making.

Being right is purely a support of how you organize your map of reality. It is not the truth; it is your truth. In forcing your right as the only right, you are reinforcing the separateness and the duality. You are saying that the way my "I" perceives it, is it. Fine. However, you are enforcing your distinction. It is your interpretation, and your interpretation by virtue of its application, is a separation into a perceived multiplicity. It is not wrong to do it that way. That's how we human beings do it. And this is my point. We make distinctions and we put our interpretation on those distinctions. We get caught, however, in thinking that our distinctions are the truth and in doing that we separate ourselves from our Self and from each other. It is the whole notion of believing in one's construct of reality as *the* construct of reality—the non-self confusing itself for the self.

Here is an example from my own life that may illuminate the problem. Once President Reagan spoke on television about the importance of maintaining an aggressive defensive posture towards the Russians. Listening, I was caught in being right about my own theory of non-aggression, due to the impact that the U.S./U.S.S.R. relations have on humanity. I was feeling self-righteous about my position and was trying to make the president wrong in order to support the rightness of my perception.

In his argument for the military posture, the president asserted his position as being practical and accurate in light of the world situation. My difficulty was that I was seeing each of us as different, as antagonists. I thought that I was concerned for humanity and he was not.

What opened my eyes was the realization that I was arguing to make him wrong by thinking that a separate intent existed between the two of us. I never thought that it could be another way. When I let go of having all the answers, I acknowledged that from his point of view he was saying what he thought was right. He had his reasons for thinking he was right—reasons that worked in his map of reality.

My perception of his map and that of other world leaders, was that they had the mentality of tribal chiefs. Historically speaking, human beings have organized their social experiences with each other in such a manner that one must protect one's property and community against the greed and wrong-doing of neighboring communities. It has been the role and responsibility of the leader to protect the boundaries and well-being of the community against aggressive behavior, both externally and internally. It has been this way throughout recorded history. Based on historical data, Mr. Reagan's content says that it is important to maintain a strong military base. Using that information in the tribal chief context, he is right. What I was doing was holding my point of view and ignoring his perspective. I do not agree with his perspective, but it is one of the points of view strongly supported by history.

My realization completely changed how I heard what he was saying. I stopped trying to be right and started listening. It did not require my agreement in order to hear what he had to say, but in my willingness to hear him, a solution for an outcome of a united planet could be achieved.

The first level in communication is to acknowledge and honor the formation of the personality that is before you. Out of that you can develop an apprecia- for the other's point of view. One does not have to accept another's position to understand it, but by suspending the bias to hear only what one wants and needs to hear, solutions begin to coincide with desired outcomes.

The Strategy of Paranoia

The second strategy is paranoia. There is no pleasing or comforting the one who employs it. Typically the person is very bright and aware that he is so. Yet he feels insecure about his position and acts out of that insecurity. Self-preservation is the modus operandi of this life generated out of the milieu of maintaining his position.

I once had a client who was president of her own company. Her company was experiencing sporadic and mediocre success. In a brainstorming session we were exploring ideas to find what in her was impeding the development of her company. In the questioning, I uncovered her use of this second strategy—paranoia. In her hiring practices she was afraid to hire anyone who was as bright as, or brighter than, she. As a result the quality of people hired and the fruits of their work bred mediocrity.

At first she was resistant to hear this injunction, and then surprised to know that she would hold such an attitude. She finally acknowledged that indeed she sought out only those that she was superior to, but was embarrassed that I knew. Once she accepted her fear of not being in control, and was willing to explore being creatively out of control, she went on to hire people who excelled in their area of expertise, and became a leader of a team of professionals.

Another time I was having lunch with a different client. She invited me to lunch to discuss an innovative idea in education. At the conclusion of the meal the waiter placed the check before me. She became very annoyed, and expressed the thought that his presumption that I would pay the bill because I was a man was related to why she and other women had difficulty in being successful in the world. I pointed out to her that she was extraordinarily bright and had the knowledge and behavior to be very successful. I went on to tell her that her difficulty lay in her presupposition of her status. I suggested that at her level of intelligence, there was no reason not to do well. She was simply taking the edge off by having this excuse ready to apply to every situation of possible failure, thus holding an unconscious reason not to apply herself.

The Strategy of Complacency

The third strategy is associated with complacency. Those who employ this strategy think that they have arrived. They look at what they have done and feel satisfied that they have the answers. There is no need to look any farther.

I know a famous minister who is the head of a large and prosperous congregation. His church is very wealthy and successful. It is quite obvious that he knows how to manage the material side of life, and obvious, through his sermons, that he thinks he has mastered the spiritual side as well. He is smugly complacent and has the world on a string.

He is cutting himself off from growth because he feels there is nothing else for him to know. His strategy will create an eventual dissatisfaction later in life when he is looking for meaning. For this he will need contentment, not satisfaction.

The Strategy of Laziness

The fourth strategy is laziness, as when one is in a lethargic state, asleep, caught in habit. Habit is associated with the way thought organizes memories. These memories are then organized or reorganized in a way that supports one's perception of reality. Enmeshed in the patterns that one creates, one becomes a prisoner to the rhythms of the past.

In the following diagram we see the continuum of time represented by line AB, and different segments of time represented by divisions T_1, T_2, etc. A parade of events is marked a, b, c, and so forth. For our analogy, each event corresponds to a time framework. Any event has no value unto itself other than that which the perceiver assigns it. What we have then in event "a" is that it is presented, leaving open a vast number of interpretations.

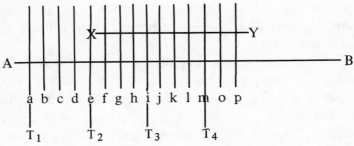

For example, if a loved one smiles at Joel, the beloved, the smiling of itself has no value. The value is assigned in the mind. The loved one has projected her smile out of her feeling, which she lends to the meaning of the smile. When Joel sees the smile, he then translates it according to the way he personally organizes reality. He may think, "She loves me," or "She is only smiling to be nice," or "She is smiling because she is annoyed," or "She is amorous," or "She is maternal," or "What does she want?" There are a vast number of interpretations available for the smile. The beloved's history will choose a range of interpretations, focusing specifically on one. He will then behave towards the loved one as if that were indeed what she was meaning in her smile. The choices in the analogy are associated with the continuity and integrity of his ego. So it goes with each event b, c, d, and so on. Each event happened in time. The perceiver interpreted the event and lent value to it.

The mind has a facility of memory (not allowing that which has been experienced to escape). Each of the events and the subsequent choices are stored in the mind. These choices are remembered in a cluster that supports the self-image. A pattern is perceived in recollection (see line XY), and accepted as one's history. This history is seen as one's self, so that when it is spoken of, it is spoken of as "I." The history has been personified and then used as a reference point to generate future decisions. Difficulty arises when the pattern compulsively dictates current and future choices.

When one does not choose the present behavior in the present and instead lets the past make all of the choices, one is referred to as lazy. This laziness causes slavery. Instead of meeting event "p" fresh and with the possibility of being confused and unprotected, one meets it the same as "m," "n," and "o."

For example, Joel automatically reached into the safety of his history for a way to interpret event "p." It was as if he went to the morgue (the storehouse of past impressions), pulled out a slab with all the corpses of his memories, reinvested them with life through his interest, and asked the corpse of "Aunt Agnes" her opinion of event "p." She gives her opinion, voice cracking, in accordance with her place in the continuum and momentum established through line XY.

Another example is driving a speedboat across a lake by looking backwards at the wake in order to steer the boat forward. It would be interesting to note the surprise of various drivers on the lake when they run aground or collide one with the other.

It is also considered lethargic to look for an answer that will truly work every time. One will eventually find that there is no answer that works every time, even for similar situations. Individuals who employ the strategy of laziness do not have the willingness to perceive that the reason their life is going the way it is, is because they are making choices to constantly create line XY. They blame outside agents for their life and do not take responsibility for it being the way it is.

The Strategy of Poor Me

The fifth strategy is "poor me," the victim. The people who utilize this strategy have an appetite and desire for many things but they do not know how to allow themselves to have anything but pain, frustration, and misuse. They want much, and feel that they have a great capacity, but they do not recognize, receive, or assimilate what they ask for. They are then unwilling to, and/or do not know how to, take responsibility for their lack, and so blame others for their pain. Like the users of the previous strategy, they cannot see how they create life the way it is.

For example, a student of mine wanted much from life materially, emotionally, and spiritually. His life, however, was not producing the outcomes that he wanted. At the same time he was jealous of another student who did indeed have what he wanted. Three things were strangling him and preventing him from being able to swallow and assimilate what he wanted. First he had an unconscious rule that said it was wrong to have those things because only selfish, bad people had them. Secondly, he did not know how to hold within his mind and lifestyle what he wanted. He knew how not to have, so that if he did get more, he would have created more "not having" in order to get rid of the abundance he already had. Thirdly, he was not willing for anyone else to have what he wanted. He thus cut himself off on an unconscious level and decreased the probability of his being able to hold what he wanted in his life for himself.

The Strategy of Anger

The sixth strategy is the strategy of anger. This strategy chooses to devour others with hostility. One using this strategy has an aggressive posture, with the intent of consuming or burning others with his rage. Whenever anything is seen as challenging his self-image, anger is used to squelch that which is perceived as antagonistic.

A friend of mine was very beautiful within and without. If thwarted, however, she would use anger associated with rejection specifically against those she loved the most. The anger ate away at her and eventually consumed her. She no longer existed, but became an "angry person." The anger within her began to seek victims and it was as if she were being driven to find them.

It is interesting to observe this strategy. Often one can find these individuals joining causes in order to be against something and take their vehemence out on a group at large. Anger is no longer a choice for those consumed by this strategy. The choice of being angry was made long ago and now they appear to be victims of an unseen force.

This last may very well be the most difficult of the strategies to perceive within oneself and transcend because there is such an investment in making others wrong. This strategy is one of the most crippling positions to hold because one refuses to see himself as contributing to the wrongness of the situation.

5
The Mind in
Yoga Therapy

Sages have, even through the present, served those in their charge by applying an entire body of knowledge for the illumination of their students. The soul, on its path of evolution to an awakened state, requires an assimilation of, and a marriage with, the other-than-conscious mind. It is this union of the two dimensions that gives a seeker the genius essential to foster the spiritual quest. At any given time one specific approach may be more appropriate and impactful than another. However, at some point, that specific practice is transcended, and is no longer appropriate as a central focus of growth because the individual has assimilated it.

My spiritual teacher once said to me, "We are already divine; we must now become human." In the attempt to assist clients in becoming fully human, I apply the multitudinous teachings and understandings of these ancient systems in the therapeutic setting.

The following sections will be an explanation of some of the principles that underlie the components of the holistic therapy that has been in use for centuries. It has been my privilege for many years to study with one who embodies these principles. Under his hand I have experienced the therapeutic approaches of the systems of yoga, and have made them part of myself. Now when I sit with a client the ancient teachings serve as the matrix out of which insights and applications surface. This tradition, in combination with conventional Western techniques of intervention, creates an interesting whole that proves to be intelligible to the client and expansive for both of us.

My conviction is that success in dealing with the client can only be born of one's own transformation. Any therapeutic progress experienced by a therapist is derived from the insight established out of who the therapist has become as a result of self-study. The commitment to continual self-knowledge is essential for the therapist. It is this commitment that brings an excitement to the relationship of therapist and client.

Yoga and Modern Therapy

Yoga is fundamentally different from historical, Western therapy models. Yoga presumes a level of psychological health and ego strength, whereas conventional therapy presumes disease. It is the presumption of health and the presumption of disease that creates the contexts of these two models out of which the various types of content can be invented.

In yoga these types of content would be: waking up to the fact that the reality is within you; that the inner and outer experiences of reality are limbs from the same tree; and that after assimilation, one is to become independent of each level of development. In modern therapy types of content would be: something is wrong which must be corrected; forces outside of you are making you do something; you have a problem, and there is a right answer to it. Because the initial presumption of therapy is invented out of the context of illness, we must, at some point, transcend this context to achieve our therapeutic goals.

In yoga we have an exploration into a "waking up" process. The sages devised practical teachings that make the seeker aware of the potentials that are in the mind but outside of awareness. Techniques have been devised by them to assist the seeker in gaining freedom. This freedom is achieved through what is called an expansion of the mind. The term, "expansion of the mind" is more about the expansion of the awareness of the mind than of the mind itself, because the mind is already in potential everywhere that "that which can be known" exists.

The masters' teachings were very pointed. Their techniques revolved around inspiring students to assimilate the teachings by incorporating the lessons into their lives.

To explain, let me first outline what is considered to be the mind from the yogic viewpoint. The word "mind" comes from the Sanskrit verb *man* which means "to think." For the sake of clarity, let us divide the mind into four functions: conscious mind, ego, discrimination, and memory.

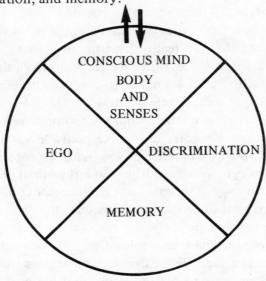

Though the mind does not possess these rigid, clear-cut distinctions, each segment is a delineation of the quality predominant in that area. For instance, in the conscious mind, conscious behavior predominates in interaction with the world, yet ego, discrimination, and memory quite apparently are also resident in conscious behavior.

The conscious mind is seen as the importer and exporter of sense impressions. The cognitive senses of smell, taste, sight, touch, and hearing go out and import the external world back to the mind as sense impressions. The active senses of elimination, procreation, locomotion, grasping, and speech export responses from the inner portions of the mind.

Next, the ego functions as the I-maker. It does so

by affirming that which it is, as well as that which it is not. It declares the self-image through affirmation and negation. "I am male" infers that I am all that I associate with being male as well as inferring that I am not female. "I am thirty-nine" infers that I am all that I associate with being thirty-nine as well as inferring that I am not any other age.

Next, discrimination organizes, sorts, and judges all information. It has two sides—the digital, rational, left brain function, and the holistic, intuitive, right brain function.

Last, there is memory, the storehouse of all past sense impressions. Conscience, or the subjective storehouse of merits and demerits, is the principle through which one selects specific responses to any pending actions.

The conscious mind, via the senses, perceives according to their tuning sensitivity. An important point must be made here. The senses predispose a certain type of experience called human. We perceive according to our humanness and not according to an absolute reality. Another way to say this is that our humanness interprets because of the types of perception that are available.

The reason reality is the way it is, is because humans construct it that way. A human being in a circumstance will experience only the human qualities of the circumstance because the sense receptors are tuned to picking up only certain kinds of data.

Some of you may be familiar with the question: When a tree falls in the forest and there is no one there to hear it, does it make a sound? This is also posed in the classical limerick:

There was a young man who said, "God,
I find it exceedingly odd
That a tree, as a tree, simply ceases to be
When there's no one around in the quad."

And God answers:

"Young man, your astonishment's odd
I'm always around in the quad.
For the tree as a tree never ceases to be
Since observed by yours faithfully, God."

Obviously when the tree falls, it disturbs the air and the ground beneath it. If there is an ear to be affected by these vibrations, the vibrations will be interpreted by the human ear as sound. Thus the sound of it exists in the human ear. In the same way, the light of the sun exists because humans have eyes.

To show the working of this model, let us say that an event takes place which we will arbitrarily label "yellow." So we have a yellow event that is interpreted by the conscious mind in the context of its human boundaries. The yellow event is delivered to the next stage in the mind process, the ego. At this stage the ego identifies or not with the incoming yellow data. I equate the ego with a board of directors. Let us say that our board of directors is predominantly blue. It will tend to see everything as blue. So the yellow event is delivered to the mind, and the board of directors will either not see it at all (because, after all, it's not blue), or it will filter yellow through its blueness, with the end product being a green event.

The green event is now delivered to the discriminative faculty. The discriminative faculty judges the green information and translates it into mind language. The memory receives the green data input. It scans its data bank to find what would be, based on history, the most appropriate response to green data.

Let us say memory comes up with a red response. It sends back to the discriminative faculty the red response which discrimination will then propose to the board. The board will not have it, because it does not want the outside world to know that it has those kinds of responses to these kinds of events. It will either reject or table the proposal, not allowing the response to be expressed, or it will modify the response and filter it through its blueness, thus delivering a purple response for the conscious mind to export.

This is how confusion is bred into the mind or delivered to the world. Yellow in, purple out! I am sure that some of you have experienced delivering a communication to someone and the feedback that you got from them did not even remotely resemble what you had originally said. This is confusing for the discriminative and memory faculties, and most probably confusing for whoever delivered the yellow communication.

A point must be made here that the unconscious faculties of the mind do indeed receive the yellow information. It is the ego or the board of directors who operate only with what they choose to see and pass on.

Yoga practice at the beginning is designed to impact the board of directors. Techniques are given whereby the ego begins to acknowledge the existence of yellow and have the ability to interact with yellow in yellow terms rather than always in blue. Meditation is one of the techniques that brings about this mindfulness of a wider spectrum. The meditational mindfulness can, in this instance, be described by the following metaphor.

You are sitting quietly, experiencing your personality as you explore the inner dimensions of your mind. The board of directors of your mind is the dominant factor of your personality that tends to influence in a major way all of your decisions. You are in the board room, and the board is seated. Hovering around the board are other aspects of your personality. These are not yet strong enough to be in a dominant decision-making position as board members. However, they all attempt to advise and influence the board as it makes its blue decisions.

When a situation that requires personal change comes forward, you might sense yourself as having a voice on how your life goes, but your decision does not seem to carry much weight. You find yourself behaving in the same old patterns regardless of your resolve.

Your meditational practices are designed to get you a seat on the board as a member of the decision-making body. Being on the board, then, you learn how to align other members with your intention. Through this you begin to bring about transformation in decisions. You begin to vote members off of and onto the board that support the directions that you would like your corporation to take.

Eventually you become the chair of the board. Your ego is now moving according to the direction that will be the most helpful in accordance with your current level of wisdom. What you will, in effect, be doing is expanding the colors out of which the board will be able to operate.

If the mind were seen as a prism and the essential nature illuminating the mind as a white light, then the white light shining through the prism would use the prism as an opportunity to express the colors that are manifestly inherent in its own self. The prism serves the light as a mechanism that transposes the potential into a manifest reality. The ego, in its first form, knows only how to be aware of the blue light coming out of the prism. The other colors are fully manifest; they are only held out of awareness.

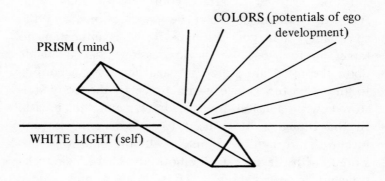

The enlightening process is the expansion of the awareness to acknowledge the existence and usage of yellow, red, and so forth, until the full spectrum made manifest through the prism is available for use. One would then have the option of receiving yellow back when yellow was sent in.

The teachings associated with bringing the awareness to light are based on a holistic model of the mind. From the yogic viewpoint, in order to bring about effective, long-lasting change, the whole of the mind must be impacted. Strategies are used to affect the physical, mental, emotional, and spiritual aspects of the mind. It is important to realize that the body is the mind in physical form. That is why it is included in the model of the mind. It is also important to realize that the spiritual side, in this instance, is what the mind perceives as being spiritual. As such, spirituality is seen as blue through the blue ego. It is not what it is; it becomes what the ego knows how to know.

As a consequence values in spirituality are determined by the color of the ego. This is why practices must be designed to affect your type of body, your types of thoughts, your type of emotions, and the spirituality that you resonate to. It is important to target all four because the impressions that are made upon the mind are stored in each category, according to the way the category functions. In the body it is stored with tension, muscle tone, and the breath. In the thoughts, it is used to access memories and invent the formation of reality. In the emotions it is stored with degrees of "emotional charge" in relationship to other events. Those with a high charge have the greatest impact upon what will be responded to in life. In the spiritual, beliefs and values predispose the entire process of body, thoughts, and emotions to receive certain kinds of information. What you believe, you will expect; and what you expect you will tend to look for. If you look for a thing you will increase the

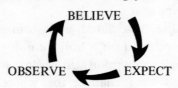

probability of finding it. And when you find what you are looking for, it will reinforce your belief that it will happen.

Defenses

The highest aspect of yoga is the ability to inhibit the mind from taking on qualities of its environment. When that ability is achieved, the self is established in its own fundamental and essential form. The sages go on to say that when this is not the case (when the mind does take on qualities of its environment) there is identification with the things that the mind is taking on *(Yoga Sutras, I.2-3)*. An example of this taking on process on a very simplistic level is delineated in the following story.

Several years ago my family and a few friends were taking the pleasure of inner-tubing down the Apple River in Wisconsin. Many people float down this river on inflated inner tubes as a form of recreation. My younger son, Ananda, at the time was five years old. He and I were floating face down on our inner tubes next to each other. We were gazing at the bottom of the shallow river pretending to be "Super Friends" flying through the air over mountain tops which were construed out of the stones on the clear river bottom. Our hands were joined so that we would not drift apart while we played the game of rescuing people. I was thoroughly delighted, and exclaimed to him, "Gee, Ananda, isn't this great? Here we are floating down the river. . . " He interrupted me and said, "Daddy, we're not floating down the river; the inner tubes are."

Thus my point. I had done the same identification at this level that the mind does at all levels. I had identified myself with the qualities of my environment, the thing that I was doing. Quite apparently the inner tube was floating down the river. I modified my humanness by riding the floating inner tube. My nature lies in my capacity to impose my sense of order, and to borrow qualities and skills from the environment. The inner tube does not have that capacity, but does have the capacity to float very easily. By identifying myself with the inner tube, I was choosing to be limited to the capacities of the inner tube—floating.

Continuing the analogy, this choice put my human ability to acquire capacities from the environment into my unconscious, and thus out of access. If by chance I would have gotten tangled in any of the fallen trees along the shore, I would have been able to entertain options for gaining my freedom based only on my inner-tubeness rather than my humanness. After modification there is a high tendency to become identified with that by which one modifies oneself and thus suffer the limitations of the identified form.

This is where defenses come into being. The mind becomes identified with the thing that it assimilates. Calling the identified state itself, it leaves everything else as "other." When there is an other, the individual self reaches out to sense what that other is. In doing so this self forms an opinion about the other and determines a behavior toward the other considered to be appropriate. In forming an opinion the opinioning itself is a subtle wall. The opinion is made in reference to what needs to be done to ensure the survival of the organism.

Due to memory, a series of these sensings gradually evolves into a history, creating a sense of continuity.

Out of this memory the I is born. The sense of I develops strategies to preserve itself and seek comfort. The outcome of these strategies is experienced as values motivated by basic urges seen as needs. As the many "others" are encountered by this "I," there is a continual sensing and opinion making going on. Eventually these opinions become established as if functioning under their own impetus. These opinions become barriers, walls of protection, between the I and all others. The process itself becomes so ingrained that it disappears from view. The medium of wall building takes on a life on its own. That is to say, one begins to acquire the habit of making walls, and the wall making mentality presumes the necessity of making walls. With this as a basic assumption any decision made is based on walls.

In our growth, we begin to recognize the unconscious and automatic defense mechanisms that have come to play in our lives. We have built the walls, assigned our personality as guard, climbed inside, and thus imprisoned, have forgotten that we have built them. We have trapped the royal being of our own self within our own walls. We then feel ourselves the victim of the walls we find so mysteriously placed around us, and we invest our energy of growth in knocking them down. The very fact of acknowledging and affirming that the wall is there, places the wall before us. Pushing against the wall only makes the wall stronger, because the strength of the wall comes from our acknowledgement of it as an adversary to be overcome. The more forcefully we fight, the stronger its adversarial position becomes in our mind. Fighting defenses strengthens defenses.

It is like the story of the young man fighting the giant blocking his path. The youth, lifting the giant up, would hurl him to the ground, only to find the giant returning with renewed strength. At some point the young hero takes stock of the situation and realizes that the giant draws strength from the earth each time his contact with it is renewed. The youth subsequently holds the giant aloft from the earth, absorbing his strength, and emerges victorious.

The initial dynamics of self-unfoldment—transcending one's walls as well as the predisposition towards defensiveness—is to first cease trying to escape. There is no escape; there is no way to tear the wall down. The greater the effort, the greater the affirmation of the wall's existence and strength. Eventually we realize that the habit of building walls and defenses backfires. After ceasing to fight and press against the walls, one must study the walls of defenses, come to know their nature, and assimilate them. Through this familiarity and awareness, one can easily walk through them.

Thus, for all intents and purposes, the prison of walls ceases to exist, though in reality it ceases to exist as a barrier. This is so because the wall building tendency will remain, but the reality of it being a barrier is eliminated or diminished. Recognizing that we are strong enough to be vulnerable, we can then live a life free of wall building.

Purity

Years ago my son and I were taking an early morning walk along the Mississippi. Standing on the bank, I was musing about the polluted condition of the river. It then occurred to me that what was actually taking place was that foreign particles were suspended in the water, and that the water's quality was such that it had the ability to hold or transport whatever was placed in it. In a laboratory scientists could easily remove all the foreign particles out of a water sample, leaving water in its pristine state. So I realized that the water of the Mississippi passing before me was as pure as its original virgin state, and at no point was what it appeared to be. What it appeared to be was something other than what it actually was.

If the river were to look at itself, it would see itself as water combined with the various particles introduced into it by the cities and animals along its bank. If it were to identify with those foreign substances suspended in it, it would then refer to itself as a "polluted river."

In the process of enlightenment, the river does not get rid of the foreign substances. Rather it comes to identify its own nature without reference to, or dependence upon, the other particles that are carried along with its nature. Nothing changes other than the identification of, and with, one's selfhood. This awareness is exemplied in another story.

An American student went to Japan to study under a famous and wise Zen master. After some time he came to find out that the roshi was fond of new shoes and fine, aged saki. One time he spied the master intoxicated. The student felt personally violated and chose to leave the monastery. On his way home he had a profound revelation that caused him to book passage back to the monastery so that he could be in the presence of the master again. He understood that the master had developed habits and tastes in his many years, enjoyed them, and yet was not attached to, or limited by, the presence of these behaviors. At any time the master could, and did, put them aside and dive deep within to fathom the vastness of his being. The student realized that he was the one attached to the shoes and the saki, not the master.

As long as there is an attachment to what you do and what you do it with, you cannot experience the ecstatic state. For attachments cannot be carried into the inner chambers. If you have a piano strapped to your back and you want to leave the room, you must first untie the piano from yourself in order to gain access to the next room through the narrow passageway. It does not negate the piano from your existence; it only takes it off of your back so that you have the freedom to use it and to leave it when you want to go into an area that is not appropriate to a piano. It is like the bold proclamation on the tee-shirt of a very dear friend of mine: "Whoever has the most things when he dies wins."

A key point to note here is that in the assimilation of this knowledge, the therapist is the one who ultimately gets worked on and transformed. In order to deliver out of the base of knowledge, you must become the base of knowledge, while at the same time being willing to transcend each level of knowledge that you attain. It is critical to understand that an intellectual grasp of the knowledge as information is not adequate to allow the therapist to serve his client most effectively.

6
Steps to Transformation

The sages were realists. In the experiments that they conducted, they looked for underlying principles, existential rhythms, and patterns of nature that were observable and repetitious. They then explored how to move creatively within these patterns, becoming at one with the nature of how things actually are. They knew that these patterns were the contexts in which human existence was spawned, and that through a knowledge of the various sets that ruled human existence, they, and those they instructed, would have an opportunity to utilize the sets as tools in their path of realization.

Like a chemist, then, the individual, through an understanding of the composite nature and formulas of life, could move easily and naturally through the known.

One such law, or observable behavior of nature, is the law of karma. The word karma is often misunderstood. Karma purely means "to act." It is popularly thought to mean negative consequences catching up with one. What karma really means is that we are the architect of our destiny.

In a therapeutic setting, being clear about the nature of karma sets behavior inextricably in a frame of personal responsibility. This is ultimately empowering because in it each individual is acknowedged as the source, the creator of his circumstances.

For example, I remember how often in my life I would wait for someone else to change in order for my life to get better, thus doing nothing to transform myself. And what if they didn't change? Some people did not, and I would still be waiting to get better after they got better. I remember even feeling that I was right. I later discovered that being right can be a crippling position because it becomes self-righteousness. It ends up being an excuse to do nothing. If being right is not producing the outcomes of transformation, then I need to reevaluate my position.

The sages express karma as a rope of three strands: the strands of desire, thought, and action. Desire is housed in unconscious drives that exist as archetypal forms not yet translated into human behavior. Thought is a translation of these unconscious drives into a syntax of humanism. The organizational behavior whereby the human organism articulates itself in the grammar of its existence is action. Thus we have desire from the unconscious; thought, the organizing principle; and action, the organized behavior. Within this pattern the human being acts upon objective reality generating consequences of those actions. Those consequences are fed back to the unconscious or the other-than-conscious dimensions to satisfy the desire. Note that consequences are results and are not intrinsically negative or positive. The thoughts select and interpret the data that it will be aware of, accepting satisfaction in the interpretation. We now have the cycle: desire—thought—action—consequence—interpretation.

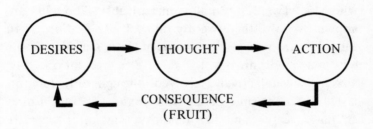

Let us interject this in life. Sarah is sitting alone in a restaurant, waiting for a business associate to meet her. She becomes self-conscious at being alone in a public place. This self-consciousness arises out of her other-than-conscious mind. It can conceivably be a generalization of the desire for connectedness, a sense of belonging. She experiences this as feeling out of place.

For our purposes we will have her personal inner resources unable to bring this feeling into harmony. Her thought processes begin to seek ways to rectify her anxiety. In her thoughts she realizes logically that there is no need to be anxious, and yet the kinesthetic experience of anxiety persists.

Unable to mentally resolve the situation, her thought process turns from an inward perspective toward the outer world in order to find resolution. It occurs to her that smoking a cigarette can be used to fill the time and assuage the feelings of anxiety. She lights a cigarette, inhales, and enjoys the response her nervous system has to the smoke. She has involved herself in the activity of locating and lighting the cigarette. She spends the next few moments relating to the cigarette much like to a companion. The whole process temporarily satisfies her need for involvement in a social setting.

Thus we have here a desire to resolve anxiety which is viewed internally unresolvable. Thoughts are applied to solve the inwardly unresolved situation. Then thoughts are generated associated with stimulating the external environment to achieve a resolution. The anxiety is subjectively resolved, though only temporarily. The next time Sarah feels anxious she again does an inner search and her memory may offer cigarette smoking as an option to be explored and acted upon. Gradually a pattern is established, becoming self-perpetuating. Whenever desire associated with anxiety appears, the probability of choosing a cigarette becomes greater. The behavior is woven into habit: desire, thought, action, consequence.

Next a process of translation takes place of which two sides exist. First, Sarah will begin to generalize the habit of cigarettes to other circumstances that prove to be immediately irreconcilable, such as emotionalism, embarrassment or impatience. She begins to associate the process with the consequence or fruit (smoking). Secondly she becomes attached to the fruit of the action and begins to focus on strategies to procure the fruits (cigarettes) so that, in this case, in addition to psychological addiction to cigarettes, a physiological addiction takes place.

This is much the same as feeling empty for whatever reason and subjectively feeling it impossible to fill that void. Food is used to numb the feeling of emptiness, physiologically creating a sense of satiation. Eventually eating oneself into oblivion is used to anesthetize the nervous system.

Through desire, thought, action, fruit of action, and the attachment to the fruit we can see how the pattern of karma is formed. The sages understood that the personality is purely a bundle of habits, and that the formation of compulsive behavior is the context out of which individual experience of reality is formed and lived.

One can transform the components of the formula of karma. Skillful action is the first teaching because this is the most tangible element of the formula for the beginner. Next the transformation of thoughts is used. Thought is the interpretation of framing of other-than-conscious urges. Change your interpretation and you change the fruits, or the consequences, because you will change the actions that you are inspired to perform. Granted, the actions or behavior can be modified, and as a consequence, so can the fruit. Yet if the thoughts are not transformed, they will create the emotional pressure that increases the probability of going back to old behavior patterns.

Next the attachment to the fruits of one's actions is targeted for transformation. The power of this step lies in the fact that if one is not attracted to the fruit, one's attraction to the pattern will decrease, empowering one to choose in the present the best course of action one knows how to choose. With the formula in hand, transformation can be brought about by 1. skillful action, 2. taking responsibility for creating what passes through the network, and 3. later taking responsibility for being attached to what passes through the network, thus becoming empowered to transform it.

Storytelling

A practical way to explain the concepts of yoga, particularly that of karma, is to tell a story about it. Throughout time sages have utilized storytelling as a medium for delivering very powerful teachings to their listeners. Models of behavior in an "as if" frame would be outlined as their tale unravelled. Masters told ancient stories, relating details of their own experience, of a wise person, a fool, or a seeker of whom they have heard. This is all metaphor to overtly (yet primarily covertly) deliver valuable information that might otherwise be forgotten.

I have watched with awe as my *gurudev* wove story after story over the years, occasionally changing the person who did the action to fit the current circumstances. It is important to know that everyone in these stories is representative of a subpersonality of ourselves. They are merely different parts of our beingness, interacting with the others. Examples of some modern storytellers are Madame Marie Von Franz, Joseph Campbell, Rudolph Bettleheim, Einrich Zimmer, and those in the Jungian school of psychology.

I utilize storytelling quite extensively in therapy settings, especially when I work with teenagers in a seminar. This ancient technique always proves to be an invaluable mechanism for delivering what is sometimes difficult and abstract material.

The following story, for example, delivers specific information about the concept of karma, which will be discussed afterwards. In a typical therapy setting, however, this condensed story would be greatly expanded.

There was once a young prince, named Prince Darling, who was given a ring by Fairy Truth when she promised the dying king to befriend the boy forever. The ring pricked his finger whenever he was bad. The power of the ring guided his rule, making the kingdom so prosperous and content that his subjects called their ruler Prince Darling the Happy.

As the years went by the prince fell under the unfortunate sway of his opportunistic foster brother and court advisors who sought favor by encouraging his conceit and selfishness. By and by Prince Darling took off his ring to be free of its painful pricks. Why should he wear it when others were applauding his greatness?

One day the prince fell in love with a beautiful peasant named Celia, and asked her to marry him. She refused. In her eyes the prince had become too wicked. His advisors appealed to his royal ego, telling him to imprison her. And so the prince committed Celia to the dungeon.

That same evening Fairy Truth appeared before him. She elaborated his misdeeds and declared that in consequence he must take on the very form of the animals whose behavior he imitated. As she spoke, Prince Darling assumed a lion's head, a bull's horns, a wolf's feet, and a snake's body. Immediately he was transported to the forest. He angrily blamed the fairy for his miserable condition. Soon he was captured by his own subjects and put in a zoo. There he began to realize his responsibility for his plight and repented of his misdeeds even though he was continually mistreated by the irascible zookeeper.

One day the zookeeper was attacked by one of the other animals. Instead of applauding the zookeeper's demise, Prince Darling wished he could come to his aid. Immediately the door to his cage flew open and he was given this opportunity. As a reward for saving the zookeeper's life, he was transformed from the monster into a little white dog.

A few days later, while taking his bread into the forest to eat, he encountered a starving girl. He gave her his own food. Later he was astounded to see Celia being dragged away by guards. He attempted to save her, but to no avail. The scene reminded him that when he was the ruler he attempted to inflict the very same fate upon her. Now he pursued Celia's attackers to the door of the Palace of Pleasure and saw her throw a dish of food out of the palace window. Prince Darling rushed to the window just as Celia closed it. Dejected, he turned to eat the food but was stopped by the maiden to whom he had given his bread. She told him that everything coming from the Palace of Pleasure was poison.

Immediately transformed into a white dove, Prince Darling flew through the palace looking for Celia. She was nowhere to be found. He searched for her over all the land, and finally found her sitting in a cave with a hermit. Overjoyed, he flew to her side and tried to express his love. The moment she realized his affection, he was turned back into the prince.

Discarding her hermit disguise, Fairy Truth blessed the two lovers and reinstated the prince as ruler of the kingdom when he sought her forgiveness.

From that day on Prince Darling, who took to wearing his ring again, ruled kindly and responsibly with Celia at his side.

Let us analyze the characters in the story. Prince Darling represents who we think we are. His counterpart is Celia. We see in his pursuit of Celia one's inner quest of the masculine to unite with the feminine side of nature. The drama is about the obstacles that provide maturation, so that when the inner union actually takes place, one's being, seen as the royal couple, has the wisdom to rightly and justly govern the kingdom of one's own self.

Fairy Truth represents the higher self, the teacher within, who acts as a guardian and provides the aspirant with tools necessary to successfully encounter, and eventually assimilate, the obstacles. The ring can be seen as the representative of conscience. When Prince Darling set up defenses against his conscience by putting his ring aside he cut his tie with truth and walled himself off from his being. He no longer had access to the higher discriminative faculty that served as a guide in his development. At that point all was lost for him.

In the story is an influential foster brother. One will notice the motif of foster relationships in many other stories, such as Cinderella and her step-sisters, Snow White and her step-mother, Hansel and Gretel and their step-mother. This motif is designed to show the main character's association with qualities that are not intrinsic to his true self, as well as the resulting influence that takes place. They are outside agents influencing the self and, by association, seeking to control and dictate behavior to their own ends. This can be equated with the addiction process or neuroses generalized into compulsions. As Prince Darling progresses, he becomes a victim of behavior that is atypical of himself and becomes identified with it. He then does not take responsibility for what he has become. He loses the favor of his creativity, Celia, because she cannot come into existence with him being identified with his current value system.   '

Through the act of misappropriating his creativity (the abduction of Celia), Prince Darling finally finishes casting the spell on himself that he has so carefully incantated. He was the creator of that monster just as he was the creator of Prince Darling the Happy. He did not want to take responsibility for creating it, so he tried to blame Fairy Truth. This is a very valuable lesson outline for the process of becoming. Whatever it is that we have become, we have, with incredible genius, created.

The story goes on to demonstrate the process of salvation. How does Prince Darling restore himself to being human and worthy once again to rule his kingdom? A model is set up in the story. First he repented and saw himself as responsible—the creator of the monster. But note, upon the acknowledgement   of his harmful deeds he was not miraculously restored to an exalted state. It took years of behavior to create the monster. At any time he could have prevented himself from becoming the monster by transforming his behavior. He would then have generated different outcomes, such as winning the favor of Celia through good deeds. He will now have to use the same process that transformed him into the monster in order to be transformed back to Prince Darling. He will now have to form a new pattern that requires continual generation of new thoughts to generate humane behaviors, and ultimately produce fruits and desires associated with becoming human again.

It is an interesting and subtle point that is next illuminated. How does one leap to the next level? Prince Darling's opportunity came when the zookeeper was attacked by an escaped animal. Prince Darling had been mistreated by the zookeeper, even though he had been repentent. During the attack, Prince Darling's first thought was that the zookeeper was getting his just deserts, but he had an opportunity to go beyond being righteous. He sacrificed his rights of vindication. A humane, if not divine, idea flamed in his mind: he would protect the zookeeper out of a sense of kindness, regardless of their history.

The zookeeper here represents both our persisting habits and the world around us. People just do not say, "OK, don't do it again." They expect us to do it again and rightly so. We have done it in the past, so they will unconsciously expect the old behavior patterns. They will treat us according to past defense mechanisms that they have built up in association with us. We must persist, however, and when given the opportunity to act out of transformed behavior, seize it.

Prince Darling sacrificed the opportunity to behave according to the old law that would be rightfully his due. This notion of being rightfully due according to the old order and making way for the new order is exemplified in two other stories. In the Bible story,

Jacob and Essau were brothers. It was time to prepare for the House of David, and Jacob was to establish that line. Essau, the older brother, by tribal law was due to inherit the qualities that were essential for Jacob's ascendence. Jacob's mother, much like the Fairy Truth, planned and assisted Jacob in receiving the birthright and the father's blessing

Another story with the same motif is Rumple-stiltskin. According to their agreement, Rumplestilt-skin was to receive the Miller's daugher's first child were she to become queen. When she did become queen, she did not want to give up her child. She guessed Rumplestiltskin's name (which means she understood his nature), and took for herself his power, and thus was able to keep her child.

So rather than accepting vindication according to the old order, Prince Darling chose to act in a more humane fashion. He chose the forgiveness and kind-ness of the new, humane order and was transformed into a dog, an apparent step up on the scale from our point of view. He achieved the reconciliation because he chose to act out of the new context of sacrifice, responsibility, and forgiveness.

Again he advanced from a dog to a white dove with the sacrifice of his bread to a starving girl, and his acknowledgment that Celia's guards were doing nothing more than he himself had intended to do.

In the transformation from a dove to a prince, Prince Darling offered himself in loving commitment to Celia, asked forgiveness from the Fairy Truth, and be-haved responsibly by wearing the ring again. He created the pain and the delight of his life, as we all do. He was totally responsible for each of the circumstances. His genius consisted in the ability to create himself in whatever manner he desired.

To think and act out of commitment, with emotional intensity, over an extended period of time produces transformation. The way in is the way out. This is so because the way of action governs human existence. It is by getting trapped in the patterns that one draws in the sand that causes one's demise. This identification with the patterns, not the patterns themselves, compulsively links one to possession and misidentification. That which at one time served, now imprisons. Liberation is purely the strategic release of attachment to the consequences or fruits of the action. We are bound to act. The first step is to act wisely, knowing that we will become what we do.

Yamas and Niyamas

An indispensable dimension of applied yoga science consists of ten recommendations for conscience formation—five restrictions and five observances.

By restrictions we mean guidelines designed to expose and thwart behavior that creates obstacles. When the profound teachings in these guidelines are understood by incorporating experiments of them in one's life, insight becomes the constant companion for the knower. Upon first observance, these restrictions (*yamas*) may very well seem like any list of shoulds and should nots, but when explored critically, free of presupposition, and at times with an iconoclastic fearlessness, interesting outcomes may delight the seeker.

The *yamas* are: non-violence, truthfulness, non-stealing, non-possessiveness and chastity. If, on the one hand the *yamas* are designed to expose and thwart behavior that proves to be an obstacle for mature emotional development, then, on the other hand, they also create a disposition of mind that is appropriate as a vehicle to express the full potential of man. The sages found that when a quality of behavior is restricted, it tends to come up even more. This fact was purposefully implemented so that the aspirant would have an opportunity to come face to face with his own obstacles.

The first *yama* is non-violence. One's tendencies towards inflicting pain immediately surface upon consciously practicing this *yama*. The injunction not to hurt others in thought, action, and speech is stressed at the beginning of this practice. But the intention is to confront and clear the tendency of hurtfulness because of the impact that it has upon oneself. This *yama* becomes powerful when the aspirant becomes clear that his own self-preservation is at hand. In order to inflict pain, one must first manufacture the pain within one's own self. It is the removal of this self-inflicting monster which is the target of the sages.

Next is truthfulness. The value of being truthful in thought, action, and speech is both the elementary and the advanced dimension of this practice. In the interim, a subtle and profound exploration of this *yama* is taken on in the exposure of one's commitment to not being with truth, that is, not being with reality as it is. The realization that the commitment to modify reality in a way that only supports the ego is a commitment to being with untruth. This insight then brings to light the value of being with "what is," and it reframes the entire perception of reality.

The next *yama* is non-stealing. The obvious tenet

to not misappropriate the property of others at gross levels is a requirement even to start this path. It is the misappropriation at subtle and causal levels that concerns us here. Its practice helps one to realize just what is actually his. We are custodians while we are here on earth, and nothing truly belongs to us. We have a responsibility to properly care for that which we take on. Children, significant others, material objects do not belong to us. To think otherwise is to take a responsibility at a level that is neither valid nor necessary. In taking on ownership rather than custodianship we hoist the pain and consideration for maintenance upon our shoulders, needlessly inflicting a burden upon ourselves. Again, we are here reminded of the tee-shirt which reads, "Whoever has the most things when he dies wins."

The next *yama* is non-possessiveness, which is associated with non-attachment. In attachment, one becomes so identified with his environment that as a consequence he becomes limited to the potency of what he has become. He loses himself because upon becoming the creation, he forgets that he is the creator. He thus relinquishes access to his full power. He becomes only male or only female. He has access to being only rich, only a parent, only angry, and so forth. When one thoroughly identifies with something and is unable to release attachment to it, one gives up access to the potency in other areas.

Chastity is the last *yama*. Each quality of existence has its own purpose. It also has the ability for others to project upon it what they think it is. As the aspirant becomes more aware, he realizes that everything has its own purpose. He communes with the purity of that purpose. The realized individual experiences the existential quality of reality and lives at the source of beingness rather than an anthropomorphized existence.

The next five observances, called *niyamas*, are qualities that one is encouraged to develop. They are: purity, contentment, *tapas*, self-study, and surrender. These qualities benefit one all the way through to the highest states. In defining these observances, one should allow them to reveal themselves rather than impose preconceptions upon them.

The first *niyama* is purity. Consider purity as an unalloyed state. In it one has the ability to do thoroughly and singularly whatever one is doing. The fabric of the mind must be undisturbed, prepared to take on the projection of whatever context it assimilates rather than distorting the images it becomes.

The second *niyama* is contentment. It points to the necessity of having a tranquil mind. One will always be seeking, yet one must have a mind that is at ease—never satisfied, but in harmony.

Next is *tapas*. This is the willingness to leap into the fire of life in order to rapidly burn away the dross. The skill gained from this *niyama* is freedom from identification with that which is burned, and the wisdom to identify only with that which is pure. Remember, purity is that which is unalloyed, not narrowed in association with a cultural notion of what is good.

The next *niyama* is self-study. The aspirant becomes increasingly aware that everything is but the understanding that we have of it; understanding is but a projection of our own self. Realizing this, the seeker is more deeply inspired to understand himself, for he knows that upon knowing himself he will finally come to know the totality of existence. In this process he will become aware of the compulsive behaviors that modify his experience of truth.

The last *niyama* is surrender. The word carries with it such significant connotation that one is reminded to let go of what he thinks the word means. My experience has been that all of the *yamas* and *niyamas* that have gone before this are but a preparation for an understanding of this one principle—surrender. It is indeed the rowing of one's boat gently down the stream, if only for the reason that that is the direction the stream is going.

A Holistic Model

According to the yoga schema, consciousness—one's true, or higher self—is the source of health and perfection. This higher self manifests in many forms: desires, thoughts, emotions, needs, urges, values, behavior (both conscious and unconscious), body, beliefs, intuition, and many other things known and unknown.

The mind, as the cognitive instrument of the higher self, can identify with any aspect of reality, thus "becoming" that reality. As discussed in chapter two, this identification can be so complete that the mind forgets its real nature, namely, the instrument of the higher self.

The purpose of yoga therapy is to reawaken the mind to its natural role. In this way, the same mind which had been the instrument of personal suffering becomes a powerful medium of transformation, unfolding, through insight, the true self once again.

The classical yoga approach to self-enfoldment states that in order to affect change on one level, the ramifications of that change must be taken into account and integrated on other levels. Thus, in order to ensure profound and long lasting transformation, the yoga schema provides a consideration for each of the facets of the human being.

The thesis of this holistic approach is that if one initiates a behavioral change in one part of the eco system, the system will attempt to return to a state of homeostasis. The pressure to return to the established norm functions mostly on an other-than-conscious level.

Sometimes people are under the impression that therapy is sabotaging their efforts at growth because of its discomfort. In actuality its apparent pain is, in part, the eco system's attempt to return to a state of comfort. In this case "comfort" is the set of learned behavior patterns that produces familiarity, and thus security. We must realize that pain, if it is familiar, could be perceived as comfortable by the mind.

For example, if one's goal is to create awareness of emotions with a client, old thought patterns will continue to reassert rationalizations of historic behavior quite logically. In doing so, the old comfort of not feeling, or the projection of certain feelings, will tend to be reasserted. The body will maintain its predisposition to respond in specific ways to stimuli, be it exaggerated response or no response at all, therefore generating a constant pressure toward habitual emotional patterns.

If one is attempting to assist a client in achieving a sense of self-esteem and it is done at an intellectual level with logical thought, the client's emotional insecurity will arise. Even when he is sleeping, the logic of this emotional insecurity will press his mind in his dreams. Accustomed to gestures of insecurity, his body will stimulate glandular flows, modify breath rhythms, and disassociate from certain areas in defensive behavior.

The yoga system has long recognized the mutual influence of mind and body. Because of its holism and thoroughness this schema is one of the rare therapy systems acknowledging the importance of transforming the body, along with other areas, for growth. This point is key to the understanding and application of the human being. Of the many things that we do, being physical is one of them, and it effects us profoundly. At minimum, if you don't feel well, you can't do well.

If a person feels angry and thinks thoughts of anger, he will have a corresponding response to anger on the physical level. Let us say it is expressed in the pelvic region. One response could be to withdraw the pelvis out of the world by rotating the pelvic girdle behind the center of gravity of the body. Another common response is to lock the anal sphincters.

If one is feeling depressed, stimulating depressed thoughts, he will have a corresponding response to the depression on the physical level. One response could be a chronic tension in the shoulders, causing the head to bow and the shoulders to stoop.

If one is emoting fear and stimulating thoughts associated with fear, he will have a corresponding response to fear on the physical level. Responses could be a folding in of the shoulders and a caving in of the chest to protect the heart at the center of the chest, thus breathing in only the upper thoracic cavity. Another physical response may be acute disruption of the digestive system.

Therapeutic strategies must be initiated to address the emotional and mental dysfunction. They will prove to little avail, however, because pressure to return to the norm will be instigated from the physical side. Strategies must be employed to realign the body so that it will be able to respond to emotions and thoughts associated with the therapeutic goals.

Imagine an individual with chest caved in, pectoral muscles constricting the chest, head bent forward, and throat constricted. He has recently achieved insight into his fear, sense of self-worth, and moroseness. He now understands the need to experience joy in his life, yet his body will tend to keep him imprisoned and not allow a deep breath to joyously stimulate the nervous system, an open throat to howl with laughter, a raising of his head to face the world. If something is not done to remove the "armoring," the constricted posture can only allow fear, inadequacy, and moroseness to pass through it.

It is important to target each aspect of the human being with a growth strategy to insure long-lasting transformation. The forthcoming sections will elaborate techniques that are designed to bring about self-knowledge through all the levels of human nature—body, thoughts, emotions, and spirit.

7
Diet

Walking into an institution of therapy, especially in the field of chemical dependency, I have repeatedly encountered the following scene: The air is heavily layered with stale cigarette smoke; a cluster of people stand around the perpetually brewing coffee machine, clutching their third or fourth cup of morning coffee; plates of sweet rolls serve as a supplement to the snacks from the colorfully-lit candy machines.

The clients (as well as the staff) of these institutions are all very well aware that to switch from their drug of choice to another addictive substance would only plunge them into an immediate abusive pattern with that substance. If they are AA trained, step school would have taught them that someone abusive of drugs will be equally abusive of alcohol. However, they do not know (and no one has told them) that they may be harmfully addicted to the socially acceptable mood-altering chemicals of nicotene, caffeine, sugar, and food additives.

Sugar and flour, for example, in their whole state are nutritive, but in their refined state put an onerous burden on the body. Refined sugar especially acts very powerfully on the body's chemical balance, impacting the emotional and rational capacities of the brain.

A friend of mine goes through dramatic mood swings and falls into a deep sleep soon after eating sugar. So severe is her condition that she has even taken naps while in a restaurant. After someone suggested she read a book on hypoglycemia, she changed her diet and has since noticed dramatic mental and emotional changes in her life in addition to an increase in energy.

Another friend has a delayed reaction to sugar. Anywhere from six to twenty-four hours after consuming sugar products her entire way of thinking undergoes a dramatic shift in response to the changed body chemistry. When sad or angry she craves sugar. She rationalizes at each use that this time will be different. Then, like the alcoholic, she thinks that one cookie is good, and two are better, and so on. Once set in motion, the craving, which comes from the resulting imbalance, requires more sweets some hours later. She reports that she begins to feel like a violin string that is wound too tight. She begins to be hypercritical due to heightened sensitivity, and experiences some paranoia associated with personal history. She then feels that people are against her, and often cannot control the accompanying intense anger. She goes through these and other lines of dysfunctional thinking born out of the chemical imbalance of a brain impacted by toxins while sincerely believing at the time that her interpretations are clear and accurate. Yet a few days after withdrawing from sugar, she again becomes gentle and easygoing.

After one such episode she reflected with me upon what took place. She said that it seemed as if she was now looking back on another person and was amazed at remembering her former behavior. Life for her, and others like her, takes on an entirely different dimension when the blood chemistry is changed. Trying to reason with her or intervene therapeutically at the time of toxicity is senseless. One would be speaking to her chemistry and dysfunction and not to her. As we have seen, the clarity that the therapist seeks cannot come into existence in a brain bathed in toxic substance. One must first restore the chemical balance in order to contact the person behind it who can see, feel, hear, and orchestrate the insight and transformation.

Orthomolecular psychiatry is a branch of psychiatry that seeks to produce a normal chemical balance in the brain with substances that are indigenous to the body. This branch of psychiatry was developed by Dr. Linus Pauling in the 1970's. Work in this field has demonstrated the connection between dysfunctional behavior and inadequate amounts of vitamin B_1, B_3, B_6, B_{12}, biotin, vitamin C, and folic acid in the brain. Amino acids and other substances are also being recognized as effecting mental and emotional behavior.

Scientific research in the field of psychosomatic medicine is emerging more and more into the limelight as a major concept in understanding the workings of health. There is mounting evidence showing that brain chemistry affects clarity of thought, emotions, and mood alterations.

The brain is surrounded by, and dependent upon, glucose (blood sugar). The brain uses the glucose for its energy needs, such as directing respiration, sense perception, thinking, and hormonal control, among many other functions. Actually the brain, which represents only 2% of the body's weight, uses more than 20% of the human organism's oxygen and 15% of the body's blood sugar. Blood sugar broken down in the brain, in interaction with appropriate vitamins and minerals, contributes to the production of chemical substances called neuro-transmitters. These transmitters are designed to carry messages across the blood-brain barrier, a membrane that isolates the brain tissue from the rest of the body in order to keep substances in the blood stream from indiscriminately entering the brain.

The brain is more dependent on proper nutritional ingredients than any other part of the body. If the transport system of biochemical messages or nutrients in the form of glucose and vitamins is not balanced or properly met, dysfunction of the ordering of the body, in addition to dysfunction of behavior, thinking, moods, and memory will be experienced. Dr. Jeffrey Bland in his book *Nutraerobics* says, "Different types of mental illness are related to serious imbalances of these various neurochemicals, and less extreme imbalances may produce behavioral and personality changes. Recent research indicates that dietary intake can lead to alterations and imbalances in these neurotransmitter substances, thereby having an impact upon brain chemistry and ultimately behavior."*

In laboratory research associated with the effects nutrients have on the brain, it is found that there is linkage between food and neurotransmitter production. If the brain needs the production of these neurotransmitters, a craving for the necessary nutrients is induced in the body. For example, there is a relationship between serotonin levels (a neurotransmitter), carbohydrate craving, and depression. Studies are currently underway to investigate the body's initiation of carbohydrate craving. The satisfaction of this craving has been found to be a natural way of generating an antidepressant mood swing.

An article in *Omni* magazine speaks of the research of Dr. Richard Wartman, a neuroendrocrinologist. Dr. Wartman has done extensive research with people who overeat and crave carbohydrates. He noted that a group of obese subjects ate balanced meals of about 1900 calories per day. Yet in snacking, they consumed an additional 1000 calories daily. When they had free access to choose between carbohydrate and protein snacks from a vending machine, they chose the carbohydrates. When asked how they felt just prior to snacking they used descriptive terms similar to those used by patients of depression.

Dr. Wartman then adds: "What do carbohydrates do for these people? Exactly what antidepressant drugs do. They increase serotonin and thereby alleviate

*Bland, Jeffrey, *Neutraerobics.* (San Francisco: Harper & Row, 1983) 107.

depression. They improve mood, diminish sensitivity to negative stimuli, and ease the way to sleep."* The question pointed to is whether a connection exists between eating disorders such as bulemia and anorexia, and serious emotional dysfunction.

Another researcher, psychobiologist Norman Rosenthal of the National Institute of Mental Health, is investigating depression during periods of less sunlight on winter days—S.A.D. (Seasonal Affective Disorder). He notes that at approximately the same time as the depression powerful cravings for carbohydrates occur in the subjects studied. Rosenthal's theory is that the lowered levels of serotonin cause depression, creating a craving for carbohydrates in order to increase serotonin levels.

The earlier stories of my two friends demonstrate the fact that hyperglycemia (high blood sugar) and hypoglycemia (low blood sugar) can dramatically interfere with proper brain functioning. The behavioral consequences of this can be seen in emotional mismanagement, depression, hyperactivity, and mood swings, to name just a few symptoms. Evidence about the hyperactive effect that sugar (a simple carbohydrate) has on some children is virtually common knowledge now. But it is necessary for us to realize that sugar has the same effect in many adults.

In one study of patients with mental and emotional problems, 70% of those who had been diagnosed as schizophrenic exhibited some form of hypoglycemia, as did many neurotics.†

* Kagan, Daniel, "Brain Foods: Diets that Sharpen the Mind," in *Omni*, May, 1985, p. 40.
† Hawkins, B. and Pauling, L. (ed) *Orthomolecular Psychiatry* (San Francisco: W. H. Freeman, 1973), 449.

YES International Publishers

Books for Self-Transformation

Post Office Box 75032
Saint Paul, Minnesota 55175-0032

If you would like to receive a copy of our latest YES Books Catalog and be on our mailing list for future publications please fill in this card and return it to us.
If you would like to receive information about seminars and workshops sponsored by YES, check here. ( )

PLEASE PRINT

Name..

Address...

....
City,
State..

Zip.........................

Evidence points toward a relatedness between sugar sensitiveness and alcoholism as well. In an interview, Ms. Jane Matthews-Larson, founder of the Health Recovery Center in Minneapolis, says that "Alcoholics have a peculiar genetic defect that causes their body to metabolize alcohol into a highly addictive, morphine-like substance called tetrahydroisoquinoline, or THIQ. Most alcoholics also develop hypoglycemia. . . they crave alcohol and sugar in any form, but both substances put them on a physical and emotional rollercoaster. . . ."* She says that alcohol changes the climate of the brain and that this change results in anxiety and confusion, generating symptoms usually called emotional. She goes on to state that alcoholism is thus rooted in one's chemistry and not one's personality. Similarly, Dr. Roger Williams, nutritional pioneer at the University of Texas, says that glutamine (an amino acid) and vitamin B reduce the craving for alcohol.

In spite of such data, very few drug treatment facilities use nutrition as an integral part of rehabilitation. The centers that are using nutrition realize the invaluable aid of analyzing the biochemical factors involved in the disease of alcoholism. They believe that the alcoholic may be suffering from a physical disease associated with toxicity and sugar sensitiveness, and that these must be seriously addressed in a continuum of health and recovery care.

One such program is the Health Recovery Center run by Ms. Matthews-Larson. It recognizes the close tie between diet and alcoholism, and feels that one's

* Interview with Jane Matthews-Larson in *Prevention*, Aug. 3, 1973, 98.

chances of staying dry are increased when whole grain, fresh produce, and vitamin supplements are the mainstay of the diet along with the discontinuation of harmful addictions to nicotine, coffee, and sugar. The center analyzes hair for nutrient deficiencies and toxic metal buildup, and tests blood sugar levels for hypoglycemia. They also test for food allergies in order to locate any other hidden reactions that are nutritionally based.

The center's record is phenominal. The blend of biochemical therapy and emotional support has generated an abstinance rate of 84% with great emotional improvement. This study was done over a three-year period in a follow-up program where 88% completed the program and 94% of the graduates were contacted.* This is compared to traditional drug treatment centers' abstinance rate of 35% after one year and an NIAAA study of 28% rate at four years.†

Another center for holistic health care that is very purposeful about its nutritional dimensions is the Combined Therapy Program of the Himalayan International Institute of Honesdale, Pennsylvania. There, a holistic program of health care is employed for people who want to receive individual guidance and professional help in all dimensions of their life. During the minimal two-week stay a person's diet is closely controlled and individually selected. This is combined with biofeedback training, counseling, breathing, postures,

---

* Brochure of the Health Recovery Center of Minneapolis, Minnesota.
† "The Course of Alcoholism: 4 Years After Treatment" by the Rand Corporation No. R 2433-NIAAA. Prepared for the National Institute on Alcohol Abuse and Alcoholism by J. Michael Poligh, David J. Armor, and Harriet B. Braiker.

meditation, outside exercise, and nutrition/cooking classes all under a physician's supervision in conjunction with yoga therapists. The Combined Therapy Program deals with those experiencing some mild emotional dysfunction and/or previous chemical dependency, with the largest part of their patient population being those who have no presenting problem but want to reestablish a general sense of health within themselves. Dr. Rudolph Ballentine, who heads the program, has written an excellent book entitled *Diet and Nutrition.* In addition to extensive information on nutrition, it gives some sound guidelines on diet that would prove to be invaluable in structuring a holistic treatment program.

We have already pointed out the deleterious effect of alcohol in the body. Drug abuse is often coupled with this abuse of alcohol. Yet many people feel relieved when they find that their children are not using mood-altering substances such as marijuana, but are engaged "only" in the drinking of alcohol. It is incorrect to assume that alcohol is somehow better than substances such as marijuana. Alcohol is socially acceptable—that is where the line ends. The abuse of alcohol and the abuse of marijuana create malfunction in the system. Some people are able to responsibly use these two substances, although science has not yet determined conclusively the reason why some can and others cannot.

In my counseling work I have often come across people who will use sugar, food, mood-altering substances, or alcohol when they feel stress. If this option is employed often enough, it will effect the level of toxicity in the body to the point where the brain will begin to dysfunction in terms of decision making.

Stress will be a trigger to seek the mood swing that the drug can provide. In addition to eventually needing to "get high" to stay normal, thus changing the body's chemical balance, the emotional issues anesthetized out of existence will stack up outside of awareness, creating an internal pressure for resolution. When this pressure is coupled with the unclear thinking of the toxified brain, the result is a high probability for emotional mismanagement.

So it is not only the use of alcohol or sugar that requires a rebalance of body chemistry, but the use of any substance that proves to generate toxicity. A nutritive dimension must be incorporated in therapy to help in reinstating the client into a condition of well-being.

The Yoga View

Yogis have traditionally emphasized that there are two vital processes in the body: one is nourishment and the other cleansing. They point out that these must both function in coordination with each other, and if not, will throw each other out of kilter. If the diet is toxic it will overtax the cleansing system. If the cleansing system is not adequately functioning, nutrients will not be taken into the digestive system for use. Swami Rama says that in the yogic view nourishing and cleansing are inseparable twins. Eating without properly removing toxic wastes denegrates the nutritive value of the prospective nourishing food.*

* Swami Rama, *A Practical Guide to Holistic Health.* (Honesdale, PA: Himalayan Press, 1978).

Cleansing

The imperative value of ridding the body of toxins is an ancient view in yoga. Vast numbers of cleansing practices were devised to keep the chemistry of the body in as conducive a state as possible to promote the higher functions of the brain. Attention thus was placed on the four systems that clean the body, namely, the lungs, bowels, pores, and kidneys

The yogis view the lungs as the most important excretive system of the body. This is to emphasize the brain damage that can occur if the lungs are not ventilating and removing toxins out of the blood cells as they should.

The bowels pass toxins out of the body by way of the intestines. Therefore it is important to eat a diet composed of whole foods that provide roughage to assist the body in elimination. It is recommended that one establish the habit of a bowel movement each day, the first thing in the morning, before ingesting any food. This is a yogic injunction, although doctors do not agree upon a standard for a specific number of movements per day. The emptying of the bowels is very important for health, and attention should be paid to it. Reading or any other distractive behavior takes the mind off the task at hand and does not help to promote proper elimination. As an aid in early morning elimination, the following prescription is given: Take a glass of boiled water, combine it with the juice of a lemon and a pinch of salt, and drink the solution upon arising.

The skin is the largest organ of the body and has its own cleansing process. This is perspiration. Perspiration is very necessary, and to stop its function with artificial means severely hampers a very vital detoxifying function of the body. All the skin requires to aid this process is cleansing with soap and water.

The kidneys are also essential for flushing toxins out of the body. A proper quantity of water should therefore be drunk each day to help the kidneys perform their function properly. According to the Himalayan Institute, the drinking of whey proves to be very helpful in some disorders associated with the kidneys. Whey is the liquid that remains when lemon juice is added to boiling milk, the milk solids forming cheese. Salt is one of the chief enemies of the kidneys and should be used minimally for good health.

The liver, too, plays a powerful role in one's personal emotional environment. Of the many tasks of the liver, the removal of toxins from the body is one of the most important. If the liver is not functioning properly, and does not adequately detoxify the body, the toxins will be recirculated to adversely affect the nervous system and the brain. Because of the deleterious effect alcohol has on the liver, liver damage should be suspected and investigated as a contributing factor to emotional dysfunction as a matter of course in any alcohol-treatment setting.

Nourishment

The sages were not preoccupied with eating, yet they understood the impact that nourishing the body had upon their minds. When they ate, they ate in an undisturbed atmosphere and, (though it is beyond the scope of this book), I would like to add that they were very mindful of who cooked their food and the manner in which it was cooked. If there was any disturbance while they were taking food, they would stop eating, since they were well aware of the effect that emotional upset has upon digestion.

In the autonomic nervous system, the parasympathetic branch is associated with digestion. When the nervous system gets upset, however, the sympathetic branch becomes predominant while the parasympathetic branch is suppressed. This stops digestion and routes the blood away from the digestive organs, causing the food to sit in the stomach and intestines, becoming toxic.

The yogis did not go to extremes with their food; they ate neither too little nor too much. They believed in regulating life reasonably. Food was divided into three classes according to the result produced in the body. One class of food was considered to be conducive to the refined pursuits of the mind. The second class was considered to be conducive to an active, more outgoing type of life. And the third class of food was considered to support lethargy and toxicity. They involved themselves totally with the first class or with a mixture of the first and second classes.

The first class of foods are those which are fresh, whole, natural, of high quality, not highly spiced, with neither overcooked dishes nor an excess of raw ingredients. Such foods helped one to be calm, serene, and balanced.

The second class of foods are stimulants, and are used for strength and activity. They include coffee, tea, rich sauces, highly spiced dishes, and foods that are designed to be extraordinarily appealing to the palate.

The third class of foods are those that have low nutritive value and are considered to be dead. They induce high levels of toxicity in the body. Spoiled food, stale food, low grades of alcoholic beverages, processed foods, and those heavily fried in fat fall into this category.*

For the past two years a committee of nine scientists has reviewed the latest evidence on food and nutrition for the government in order to update the 1980 guidelines of the Departments of Agriculture and Health and Human Services. The guidelines are directed at people who are already healthy and do not currently need special diets. They are:

1. Eat a variety of foods.
2. Maintain a reasonable weight.
3. Avoid too much fat, saturated fat, and cholesterol.
4. Eat foods with adequate starch and fiber.
5. Avoid too much sugar.
6. Avoid too much sodium.
7. If you drink alcohol, do so in moderation.
8. Exercise in moderation.†

What, then, would be a perfect diet? In his above-mentioned book, Dr. Ballentine has devised a universal diet designed for good health, which is flexible enough to meet individual needs and tastes. He based his recommendations upon the traditional rules of food selection from many world cultures. Whole grains constitute the main part of this diet, with beans and legumes amounting to about half the bulk of the grains. Fresh vegetables are next, in an amount between that of the grains and legumes. The fourth group is the B_{12} group which

---

* More information on this topic can be drawn from Rudolph Ballentine, *Diet and Nutrition.* (Honesdale, PA: Himalayan Press, 1976) 279ff.
† Stern, Judith, "Eating for Health," *Vogue*, July, 1985, 72-74.

includes meat, dairy products, eggs, fish, fowl, and tofu. This constitutes the smallest group of daily needed foods. The last group is raw foods, which is larger than the B_{12} group but smaller than the vegetable group. It would include raw fruit and salads. The proportion of food in this diet tends to give the most energy to the body while maintaining good health.

The yogic sages did not come to food from a position of dysfunction. Their literature on food is directed out of the intention to affect the physical, emotional, mental, and spiritual dimensions of the human being. Diet was seen in light of prevention and in terms of maintenance. Their injunction is to be reasonable with diet, and to realize that each person's metabolism and needs for nourishment are somewhat unique unto himself.

As one must have a healthy mind to communicate with one's body, so must one have a healthy body with which to express oneself—a body capable of expressing what it is to be human. It is not that a change in diet or massive doses of nutritive supplements should be applied in all cases. It is, however, because of the impact nutrition has on behavior, that this facet of human life must be analyzed in conjunction with the other dimensions of health care. With this in mind, and from the holistic view, it is vital that along with counseling, body work, breathing, and meditation, diet and body chemistry be included in the package of therapeutic intervention.

8
Body Work

The sages who developed the system of hatha yoga around the sixth century, B.C., did so because they realized that the body served as a major instrument for the spiritual development of the aspirants under their direction. By understanding the context out of which the use of hatha yoga arose, we can appreciate the genius of the systems they developed. All methods of transformation must initially, and well into advanced stages, acknowledge one of the primary contexts out of which development takes place. That context is called human being. It is the starting point of self-transformation.

This is exemplified in the story told to me by my colleague, Dr. Justin O'Brien. He was lecturing at Oxford University last year, and during the course of his work met a professor who had just returned from Africa. The professor had been invited to visit a friend who lived on a large ranch in Kenya. Upon landing at the airport, the professor was unable to find his friend, but was approached instead by a stranger who introduced himself as a neighboring rancher. Their mutual friend had requested that he receive the professor at the airport and drive him to the ranch, which was some distance away.

They collected the bags and drove off into the bush. After three hours of driving, the sun was beginning to set when they stopped at a clearing where a Travelall vehicle was parked. The rancher announced that the vehicle was for the professor's use since he himself had to return to his own ranch some miles in the other direction. He apologized for the inconvenience, but assured the professor that every care was taken that he would have no trouble reaching his final destination: the vehicle was gassed and ready; the tires were full, and there was a spare; a gallon of water was stored in the trunk; and a map of the criss-cross of trails and roads was located in the glove compartment, with the final destination clearly circled in red.

The two men bid each other goodbye, and the professor watched his new friend drive off into the beauty of the sunset. He happily got into his vehicle and started the motor while pulling the map into view. Horror of horrors! While the destination was clearly marked on the map, where he was, was not!

This is the position most of us find ourselves in throughout life. We know where it is we want to go, but we do not always realize where we are. We must realize that as human beings, being human is where we must start. The condition in which we human beings find ourselves is that we are embodied. Many of us deny this reality, and try to get where we are going by starting somewhere else. Let us take a look at what the embodied condition of a human being presents for us as a physiological being.

In the yoga view the body is seen as one of the demonstrations of the mind. What I look like physically is the outcome of the way my mind personally organizes the vehicle called "human body." The human body develops itself along the lines of the human mind the way iron filings align themselves along the lines of a magnetic field.

A favored simile of mine is that of two squirrels. If two squirrels were running before us now and one fell over dead, the difference between the two bodies would be that one would have a squirrel in it and one would not. The "something" that keeps organizing the food substance in such a manner that it demonstrates squirrelness would exist in only one of the bodies. When that "something" leaves, there is no longer anyone present to maintain the integrity of the various proteins, minerals, and other substances that combine to make up the animal form which we call squirrel. As a result, we will notice over the weeks that each element will return to its aggregate relationship with the minerals and other substances called soil.

My personal experience of this dynamic is related

in the following story. I was walking through the down-
town mall in Minneapolis, thinking about how the body
is shaped by the mind. I decided to conduct an experiment on the subject. I chose something easy, a state
that I considered myself to hold fairly consistently:
I determined to walk with my head, neck, and trunk
held erect. As I said, I was under the impression that I
held this posture very well, but I reminded myself to
do it anyway. After a few moments of walking, I
checked my internal dialogue (as it is my habit to do),
and remembered my experiment. The check caused me
to realize that I had forgotten it! My head was down
and I was walking to avoid making eye contact with
someone who was walking towards me. I decided,
"This is silly," and reaffirmed my part in the experiment.

The next thing I recall is that I was standing in
front of a Woolworth's window, deeply engrossed in the
Mickey Mouse lunch boxes in the display. That is
what tipped me off to my being distracted. I had no
interest whatsoever in the contents of the window, and
yet emotionally I experienced myself as being trans-
fixed. Remembering my experiment again, I cast my
gaze back along the path and realized I had turned to
the window subconsciously to avoid a man who reminded me of my military days.

Once again I determined to walk down the street
with my head up no matter what, rationalizing that I
was a yogi and ought to be able to string together more
than three seconds of concentration at a time. Low and
behold! My next internal dialog check revealed to me
yet again that I had forgotten the experiment. I had
been walking down the street meticulously avoiding

each crack on the sidewalk, reciting an old school rhyme I used to sing as a child, "Step on a crack, break your mother's back."

This time I insisted that my internal tendencies hold my head aloft and erect, but in response a notion within said that I should be more humble and not look so proud. I responded that I was not advanced enough to be humble, since I did not know what humility meant. Ahyway I would like to continue with my experiment.

This conflict arose within between my habitual, historical self and my intellectual self who was conducting the experiment. What was happening was that my experiment was forcing my mind into a state of error. That is to say, the experiment was requiring my mind to function at a level that was not usual. On a scale of 1 to 10 my self-esteem was usually at a 7. I had just thrust myself into the physical posture of an 8. My muscular-skeletal system was at ease in the developed 7 state. In my experiment I used conscious energy to raise my sternum, thrust my spine towards the front of my body, put my pelvis over my feet, chest over my pelvis, and pull my head up and out of the shoulders. At the same time there was a constant pressure in my body to return to normalcy. The conflict arose between the tug of normalcy and the pull of the experiment.

The distractions were a result of the attempts and justifications to go back to normal. The body had been molded by the mind. Over the years fascia had glued themselves together into a muscle form that my personality assumed in flesh. All of my memories and impressions told me it was not OK to hold my head so erect all the time, to keep my chest so expanded and forward all the time, to meet everything directly face on. When there are reasons not to meet life directly, a physical adjustment based on defense is made. That adjustment throws the body off of its center of gravity. A corresponding portion of the body must then make an adjustment in order to keep the body erect against the force of gravity.

The study of body language is the study of the interpretation given to the compensatory interaction of an erect body with gravity. Yoga postures are designed to restructure the muscular/skeletal system into its correct natural alignment. This puts the body into direct contact with material reality in a manner that it is designed to experience. Instead, we typically find ourselves encountering life as seen through our defenses. Our physical view is shifted off from center a few degrees resulting in a rotated pelvis, a lowered shoulder, an overdeveloped trapezious muscle, or a concave thorasic cavity. Normally we do not see or experience existential reality; we end up seeing what we see through the fetter of our senses.

In my work in therapy I use the body as a therapeutic context to create outcomes whereby other portions of the mind can be impacted. As often as possible I create an overt pattern of coordination of the body, breath, and awarenss. When these systems are coordinated, the climate for self-awareness exists both biologically and intuitively. By adding the intellect to the process we have physical, emotional, and mental components in concert. Creating harmony and synchronization in a human organism provides the opportunity for an expanded self to be invented. As a result a frame for new ideas, dreams, thoughts, and outcomes is brought into existence. The total human being in the process of becoming more human is the context in which development can take place.

Our body is our memory, our diagnostic tool, our reality check, our reference point in organizing the rush of life as we map out our experience and our interpretation of what life is. In order to do this we must first fully inhabit the bodies we create. The physical environment, the thoughts, dreams, and feelings we create must be inhabited in order to involve ourselves in our own creation. In coaching for a coordinated, synchronized, flexible system I offer a context for experiencing the responsibility for creating and expanding a map of reality—a spatial, environmental, physical, cognitive, emotional map. I am proposing to wake up and live in this map we have created so we can demonstrate what we have become through interacting with it. We can explore to our limits during our becoming, step outside of our boundaries, progress to assembling new boundaries, and then bring into existence a new, expanded map of reality to be explored.

Accessing System

One of the outcomes that I assign myself in coaching my clients is to make them familiar with how they retrieve information from their memory and the process by which they organize their personal map of reality.

In the work done by Bandler and Grinder referred to as neurolinguistics, patterns of unconscious behavior have been observed, and some of the processes by which the unconscious mind accesses its storehouse of information for conscious use have been unravelled.

Bandler and Grinder noted that human beings use the five senses externally to gather and communicate information, while also using those very same senses to communicate and gather information internally. They classified the methods as either visual (seeing), auditory (hearing), or kinesthetic (bodily sensation, taste, and smell). They classified experience as either internal or external, constructed or remembered. Internal is the class of experience associated with memory and/or current personal biological experiences; external is the class of experience associated with information coming from outside of the immediate personal system. They noticed that human beings tend to unconsciously favor access to information through one system over another.*

Many valuable techniques to interact with patterns of unconscious behavior have been devised and employed as a result of this work, and I have implemented much of it in my therapy programs. Its value in therapy lies in its ability to help a client discover his favorite system of accessing and bringing forth into awareness information previously outside of his awareness. This so informs them about the construction of their reality that they can, even at an early stage, experience dramatic stages of transformation in association with how they communicate within themselves.

In the techniques offered in subsequent chapters, the reader will notice that I occasionally suggest that the therapist ask clients how they are accessing information into their current structuring of reality. I do this much more frequently in person. In the process

*Bandler, Richard and Grinder, John, *Frogs Into Princes*. (Moab, Utah: Real People Press, 1979).

of delivering a class in postures or leading a relaxation or guided imagery I will instruct participants to notice how the information comes into their field of awareness.

Choice

One of the principal concepts in the maturation process is that of choice. In working with groups in a therapeutic setting I seek to make evident the realization that we choose the interpretation of our experience of life, the formation of our boundaries, our bodies, and our character. My intent is to propose waking up to choice rather than somnambulistically walking through life letting previous choices live life through me.

I repeatedly remind clients to choose to be here, or choose to reflect, choose to explore, or choose to employ resourceful patterns of behavior. The key is to remember to choose at each point. Wherever one is halted in the process of life is a choice point. One must then decide where to go next. One can either make a choice based on his current level of knowledge, or recoil from the choice and let his history move him in puppet-like fashion. As this remembering to choose at choice points becomes more present, additional options can be brought into play. Then skills that have been delivered in the context of therapy, peer relations, and other new perspectives can be considered along with tried and tested patterns of unconscious behavior. Unconscious boundaries once set with good intention may now only be useful on occasion rather than as the standard.

In coaching clients I am careful not to deliver my value system in terms of what should be done; I deliver instead the conscious use of the paradigm called choice.

I do not say what to choose; I only offer that they notice a choice point exists, and should remember to choose new or historical behaviors in it.

Intent

One's intent throughout life, and specifically during body work and yoga postures, is pivotal to the process of self-unfoldment. To yield the extraordinary return of this process, we intend to impact the body through physical manipulation and mindful intent. The intent is critical here because intent polarizes the interpretation of the neuromuscular responses. In this way we relate the reponses to issues of self-transformation as differentiated from other issues, or from no issue at all. Thus any sensation will be interpreted both physically as well as psychologically. During group work encouragement is given to continually organize the collective intent around transformation from both perspectives.

It is noticeable that being limber of body is not a guarantee of self-knowledge. If this were the case, most dancers and gymnasts would be in a sublime state of wisdom. Our body is one place where our serial interaction with life becomes apparent by being made flesh. Our attractions and repulsions, our identifications and fears, our becomings, how we move through time, and how we occupy space, shape our body through our interpretation of life's events as we encounter them.

Anything that pushes against our self-made boundaries stimulates other-than-conscious recollections associated with the drawing of those boundaries. This may come forward into the conscious mind and be interpreted kinesthetically as muscular tension, heat, pressure, sense of weight, shaking, or nausea. Or it might be interpreted visually as a replaying of the event, waves of color, or patterns of light. It might also be interpreted auditorially as internal dialogue with parental injunctions, logical judgements, music, buzzing, or other sounds.

Intent becomes powerful at this time. If one has the clear intention to explore one's self by examining conscious and other-than-conscious data, then when something surfaces from the unconscious it will be sensed in a holistic spectrum, and viewed as connecting to all facets of life.

This must not be done so as to cripple development by over-analyzing every bit of data that comes up, but to be done intelligently so as to acknowledge the connectedness of all things. Thus I might realize that my digestive disorder is connected to stress, that the roundness of my shoulders connects to my issues of depression, and that most likely my lower back pain is connected to my sexuality and its power. Aligning intent physically manifests an arena whereby boundaries can be examined. Then a breakdown can be viewed as an assignment to inspect one's boundaries, and decide whether they need to be reinforced or exceeded to make way for the new.

Anthropomorphizing a bodily posture makes this point clearer. For our example, let us attribute to the posterior stretch posture the qualities of a master teacher, and to the body the qualities of a student. Our intention is that the student take on and assimilate the physical qualities, as well as the behavioral responsiveness and flexibilities of the master. In this way the "beingness" of the posterior stretch will show up in the body and continue to its physical health. It will generate an environment responsive to the flow of a more complete spectrum of emotional responses. The physical body will release its current armoring against experience and open to the flexibility and ease generated by the posture.

Biases

Through many years of body work in therapeutic settings I have found it effective to employ certain biases. These biases have value in that they give me a place to start evaluation of the client. They will, of course, break down at some point. However, if this limiting factor is kept in mind, biases can be very effectively used.

For example, to say that an inability to bend at the knees is a sign of defiance is a bias. It may not be true in every case. One client may have injured his legs in an accident; another may have stiffness due to recent over-exertion in an exercise program; another may be taking medication that causes dizziness. All of these circumstances may make the bias false. Yet in most cases the bias would point out that the therapist should definitely investigate the client's issues with authority in order to help him through any dysfunctional psychological armoring. At the same time he should be assisted in increasing physical flexibility in that area of the body.

In teaching the postures I use every opportunity to point each participant to the awareness of specific experiences taking place within him auditorially kinesthetically, and visually. The use of bias then functions as a clue in examining behavior on each of these levels.

With the lead provided by a bias, one is often able to recognize typically hidden pieces of neurologically-based behavior. The discovery is designed to expand the client's individual conscious awareness into realms of the mind that are usually outside of awareness.

Since there are strong correlations from transforming the body to transformation in familial, social, and individual behavior, the client is directed to observe his bodily unconscious behavior and create linkages that translate across into family, social, and personal environments. The larger outcome is to create an appetite in him for self-awareness that he can choose to implement whenever he wishes.

In the explanations of yoga postures in the next chapter, I will share some of my biases, presuppositions, and experience on the psychological implications of the postures. I have found all of these to be accurate for the most part, and invite the reader to explore them, not as truth, but merely as information passed on to him for his own experimentation.

Introspection

When one closes one's eyes, the ability to be introspective is increased. Closing the eyes closes off the external input of one channel of involvement—the visual. Thus the distraction of translating, interpreting, and judging (oneself and others) is reduced. For this reason, during sessions of body work I instruct students to close their eyes at the end of each posture. They are guided in a process of exploration of this historically unconscious behavior. This is done with the intention to enhance living in the inner world of subjective experience as well as the outer world of external phenomena.

We are citizens of two worlds—an inner world and an outer world. The value of being awake to this fact is that one can choose to be skillful in each, knowing the impact each has on the other. One can also begin to realize that some skills are best.developed in one arena (inner or outer) with a competency check in the other.

Let us use fear to illustrate. There are yoga practices, the headstand for instance, that tend to stimulate fear in some practitioners. The practices, however, offer several choices in dealing with this emotion. The fear can be met and experienced for forty seconds while in the posture and then released, so the overt stimulation of anxiety is removed. The posture can also be worked on in the memory where the associated neurology (via the emotional stimulation) can be controlled. Or the fear can be handled in doses: tackled for forty seconds in the pose, released, and then met again for another forty-second interval, and so on, until it is resolved. In this manner the individual can enter into a less than resourceful state in controlled doses and use these periods and after as time to explore while in physical safety.

Relationships can be resolved in the outer world where movement through time and space is slow, and error can be adjusted before harmful consequences occur; or they can be worked on in the inner world employing the quickness of imagination with dreaded outcomes speedily traveling the well-worn circuitry of expectation.

It is not so much that one world is preferable to the other, but that each has its own value, its own power. We are travelers between these two worlds;

the opportunity here is to become a skillful traveler who targets development for the arena most suited for effective growth.

When this concept is grasped, another factor for self-knowledge is introduced. The postures are used to access the wealth of internal states. In performing any action, but particularly hatha postures, which are designed to sensitively explore boundaries, one can come into contact with the limits of one's performance, be it physical, mental, or emotional. These limits define one's character, one's current ego development, one's self-image. Sensations that persist after the posture is completed give access to a rich rainbow of other-than-conscious responses to what was previously experienced. These yield additional insight and an increase in body awareness. Therefore it is also of paramount importance to explore the spaces between the postures. We inhabit not only the body we have created, but also the time we have created in the form of memories stored in the body that continue to emerge long after the posture is complete. Spaces between the postures should be explored as thoroughly as are the postures themselves. Who one is shows up in those spaces.

Discrimination

One of the values that body work, specifically hatha yoga, offers in therapeutic intervention is the cultivation of the faculty of discrimination. In the yogic strategies of self-transformation, discrimination is considered to be the first cause of bondage and also the mechanism of freedom. The bondage is the inhibition of the mind by the distinctions it creates. Freedom is the realization that the distinctions are made by the mind, that these distinctions are not the self, and finally that the concept "distinction" nevertheless creates the sense of self in time and space.

The way hatha yoga can be employed as a discriminative strategy for transformation is by creating a context in which the client makes more precise distinctions, and then is coached to be responsible for having created these distinctions. The intention here is to create the opportunity for a level of cognitive excellence and then use the knowledge gained as an analogue for other systems, such as mental and emotional development in addition to personal relationships.

During a session one can highlight a particular portion of the body with the invitation to explore the sensory stimulation that is currently taking place. In a seated forward bend or a neck exercise, for example, I will suggest a conscious selective exploration of neuromuscular responses, their origins and directions, and types of kinesthetic behavior, such as heat, pressure, or motion. I will also ask if there are memories or emotions emerging as clients experience the posture and if, over the weeks, they notice the same or similar recollections associated with the same posture. To assist them in understanding how they organize reality, I will ask them to note if they favor accessing their information with pictures, with sensation, or with sound. Thus they are frequently invited to discriminate by isolating, focusing specifically on a certain muscle area, and being aware of whatever comes forward. In doing so a meta-model is illustrated that can be referred to in other systems. The model is "locate, define boundaries, notice responses." This is done with a minimum of translation or interpretation. My intention is to refer to this technique later in other dimensions of therapy.

The body is one of the forms of memory of the mind. The manner in which we interface with the world, and the reality that we map out as a consequence of our unique interface, modifies the shaping of the human form. The readiness to experience and explore what life presents will impact the development of the body by allowing it to interact with the world naturally and unimpaired. We will see a healthy, natural development throughout the whole being—physically, emotionally, mentally, and spiritually. Among many other signs and symptoms, the spine will be erect, the chest open, respiration easy and diaphragmatic. There will be a brightness of the eyes due to a balance in the autonomic nervous system, a pleasant body odor, and a quality of lightness to the frame. There will be an aura of clarity, self-assuredness, tolerance, and pleasantness of mood detected in the sweetness of breath.

When the natural development is thwarted by an unwillingness to interface with life as it is, the human organism shapes itself around a need to suppress its natural expression in life. It behaves incongruently, and is subject to the puppet-like actions of the conflicting drives in the unconscious. This is because the emerging ego, in the process of becoming independent, makes defensive adjustments in order to survive in its interaction with life. These adjustments are not a fault of the ego; they are purely an articulation of a coping mechanism—the ego's desire to survive.

To appreciate the circumstance in which the human

ego finds itself, we must take a look at the reality it faces in its place in evolution. The ego has the responsibility of preserving the organism physically and psychologically. In its primal phase, the human organism was in a stooped position with less of the body vulnerable to attack. Upon assumption of an upright stance, the role of the ego became more complex. The physical relationship to gravity became much more precarious, and vital physiological parts that are directly linked to the psyche were exposed to meet life. From a stable, relatively protected, quadriped position to an erect biped position, protection must now be given not only to its head and neck, but to its entire front— breasts, heart, abdomen, and genitals. The ego now has an even more monumental task. As life persists, the organism is now required to meet it from an entirely different perspective. The context of this position introduces issues that did not exist in an earlier stage of evolution.

In its strategies, the ego first determines how much of life it can handle at any given time. Entire realms of behavior can be withdrawn or shut down so that the ego can cope with a manageable portion of the human condition.

In shutting down a part of the physiology as a strategy for survival, the ego chooses to rigidify portions of the organism in order to decrease the stimulation in that area. For instance, the chest may be stiffened in order to protect feelings of vulnerability associated with the heart. This rigidity armors against perceived physical and psychological attack.

In therapy we will often see a modification of the human form through an asymmetrical development of the muscles. This development will be initiated by strategies of suppression or a tightening of certain bodily parts, like a child saying "No!" in order to separate itself as an act of independence. This chronic rigidifying or holding at bay will habituate tightness and lack of movement in the targeted cutoff area, and can be studied by seeing its impact upon the skeletal structure.

Let us examine three scenarios designed for your exploration in order to produce in your physiology a kinesthetic experience of what we have been saying. In each of the three scenarios, to the best of your ability, become emotionally involved and stimulated. As the emotions are awakened within you, notice where they first emerge and note their movement through your body. At some point in the scenario, I will instruct you to suppress the emotional response pattern. Your assignment then will be to prevent any further emotional response in that direction, as if I were reprimanding you or telling you that you do not have permission to experience those feelings.

At that point notice which portion of your body stops the emotion, and which portion ends up being the repository of the inhibiting behavior. When you process the responses, make sure they are neurologically based, and not linguistically based in interpretation. Feeling good, sad, or free is a linguistic interpretation of a neurological phenomenon. Your investigation is to produce information such as "heat in shoulder, pressure in lower left chest, tingling at the perineum, spongelike squeezing in the right temple, blue color in the upper left field of vision, or sound in right ear."

After each scenario dissipate any residual emotional charge with a deep exhalation, visualizing any tension or anxiety going out with the breath. Note down what your neurological responses were in the form of posture, sensations, images, or sounds.

Scenario 1

You are walking into a meeting room which is full of people you have hand-picked as a team. You have been assigned a project by an executive board, and experience a sense of confidence because you know that you are very competent to produce the requested outcome. You have done this before, and based on your past experience and mastery, you have organized a strategy that virtually insures success. As you enter the room, you are buoyed in anticipation of success.

Upon surveying your teammates, however, you notice sitting to the left of your chair someone you specifically did not invite on your team. The two of you exchange glances and the history of your incompatability flashes through your mind. You can see the project's level of efficiency and productivity diminish by at least 25% as a result of the presence of this antagonist. You find out he has been assigned to your group by the executive board, thus making it questionable whether you would be able to remove him without much political conflict.

You are angered by the person's presence. He looks you in the eye with a turn of his lips, and his mockery unveils his arrogance. Anger awakens in you even deeper. The others look at you wondering what you will do, because they know the history shared by the two of you.

It is not OK to be angry. You are a bad, bad person if you are angry. You must not show anger; you must not allow any signs of anger to show in your manner, speech, or bearing. Suppress it, and work it out later in privacy, if at all.

Scenario 2

You are very sad. You have just received news that is creating an experience bringing you close to tears. Following your need to be alone, you go into a quiet, darkened room. You close the door, and the darkness feels comforting and womblike to you. The experience of sadness begins to move in your body, and the feeling of tears is there at the brink, though not ready to flow. You hear voices in the distance and yet you feel secure in your position behind the closed door. Your mind begins to brood over the sadness, and while you reflect, the voices get louder, making you realize that they are actually coming into the room that you are occupying.

You must pull yourself together. It is not OK for people to see you saddened to this extent. I repeat, it is not OK. As you draw upon your resources and reserves, the doorknob begins to turn, and the doors swing open. You quickly right yourself, the light is turned on, and everything is OK.

Scenario 3

You enter into a gathering of people and you see someone that you care for deeply. The bond between the two of you is so profound that halfway through a sentence from either one of you, the other already knows and is giving the answer. The communications are magical. It is a joy to experience what a human relationship can be.

Your eyes meet and you begin to walk across the room to contact the person. You realize, through the responses in your nervous system, how deeply affected you are by this human being. Your mind begins to ponder "What would happen if he knew how much I cared." The thought of vulnerability frightens you and immediately brings up defensiveness. Your mechanisms of self-preservation and separateness surface. You must show him only that you care for him to an appropriate extent. You must not let him know how vulnerable you are. As you reach your hand out to his, you look him in the eye. You are there for him only to a certain extent—most assuredly not to the fullest.

* * *

At no point am I saying that you should not experience any specific emotion such as anger, sadness, excitement, love. The nervous system is designed to have the emotions pass through it. The entire physiology experiences the wave of emotion and is done with it, as the ocean is done with the wave after it passes across its surface. We differ from the ocean, however, in the sense that we can store memory of previous waves, and then develop opinions and preferences associated with those memories. We then become attached to the pleasure of certain waves and repulsed by the pain of others. We then attempt to prevent some waves from passing through us.

The conscious and unconscious effort sustained in inhibiting expression impacts our physiology, and can be read by a skilled eye in terms of the compensations that are made by our body structuring itself in the gravitational force field. This is so because muscular deviations away from the norm pull on the skeletal structure and force the organism out of balance. Compensations must then be taken to prevent the organism from loosing balance. A defiant thrust of the head may require a pelvic shift; a concavity of the chest may cause the center of gravity to move over the heels rather than the instep, or it may thrust the head forward. In like manner, a pulling back of the left side of the torso may cause the feet to point off in two different directions.

There are also neurological responses to repression. The locking of the abdomen, for example, may force the breath into the upper chest, precipating anxiety; fear may tighten the pelvic floor and create constipation; excessive sympathetic stimulation may cause digestive or eliminative disorders; excessive parasympathetic stimulation may bring about depression.

Yoga postures were designed in part with the intent to realign the human skeletal system, to normalize repressed or overstimulated glands, and resensitize the individual to nerve impulses. This is done with yoga *asanas* (postures or attitudes), breathing practices, and the cognitive practice of discrimination by isolation.

In the following schedules I will outline the use of hatha yoga as a therapeutic intervention. It is essential to treat the yogic element of any therapeutic program with the same importance, in terms of attendance, as other elements of the program, such as counseling and didactics. When treatment centers offer yoga as an elective, clients drop yoga when it begins to have its effect. It must be remembered that yoga is a wellness program designed to plunge individuals into that which impedes their self-unfoldment. Because of this I have found that people will unconsciously create reasons for not continuing, when in actuality they are experiencing the fear of their own unresolved self. To relax, for instance, allows repressed impressions to come forward into awareness. Releasing the lower back with yoga postures may restimulate experiences of low ego strength. Breathing exercises may very well place one back inside of his own emotional field.

Schedule Proposals

The following are two suggested schedules for a thirty-minute and a sixty-minute program. If ninety minutes are scheduled in a program, either place more bodywork into the segment, or increase the length of the relaxation, breathing, and meditation segments. Another suggestion is to hold each posture for a longer period, being mindful of your clients' tolerance for duration.

These programs are recommended for three to five times per week in treatment. With the longer sixty minute program, I recommend using A twice a week and B once a week. A = 45 minutes for postures, 5 minutes for first relaxation and 10 minutes for last relaxation and breathing. B = 5 minutes for first relaxation, 15 minutes for stress reduction exercises (chosen from simple bodywork such as face massage, forward bend and twist), 25 minutes cognitive materials (those related to inner exploration and congruent with your therapeutic outcome), and 15 minutes breathing and meditation. A program meeting four to five times per week can use A three times a week and B once or twice.

30 MINUTE YOGA PROGRAM

Relaxation Exercise 2 in the Corpse Pose ——— 5 min.

Forehead / Sinus / Face Massage
Shoulder Rolls
Neck Exercise
3 Solar Salutations
Half Forward Bend
Simple Cross-Legged Twist   18 min.
Shoulderstand Series
    Shoulderstand
    Plow
    Bridge
    Fish

Relaxation 2   7 min.

Complete Breath

60 MINUTE YOGA PROGRAM

Relaxation Exercise 2 in the Corpse Pose ——— 5 min.

Forehead Tension / Relaxation
Tense Right / Left Side of Face
Eye Exercise
Forehead / Sinus / Face Massage
Neck Exercises
Shoulder Rolls, Right / Left / Both
Wrist Exercise
Horizontal Stretch

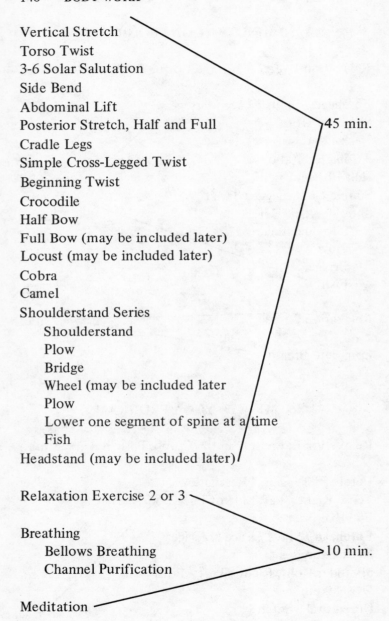

Vertical Stretch
Torso Twist
3-6 Solar Salutation
Side Bend
Abdominal Lift
Posterior Stretch, Half and Full
Cradle Legs
Simple Cross-Legged Twist
Beginning Twist
Crocodile
Half Bow
Full Bow (may be included later)
Locust (may be included later)
Cobra
Camel
Shoulderstand Series
    Shoulderstand
    Plow
    Bridge
    Wheel (may be included later
    Plow
    Lower one segment of spine at a time
    Fish
Headstand (may be included later)

45 min.

Relaxation Exercise 2 or 3

Breathing
    Bellows Breathing
    Channel Purification

10 min.

Meditation

9
Yoga
Postures

It is the intention of this chapter to describe a context whereby one can begin to discover for himself the yoga network of transformation through body, breath, and thought. This chapter has been written as a personal guide for performing and teaching the yoga postures. It can act as a criteria for the whys and wherefores of the postures, as well as an interpretation of the psychological effect that each posture evokes. I cannot recommended enough, however, that the therapist learn these postures and achieve a level of personal competency, in addition to having his postures critiqued by a competent teacher, before teaching them to others.

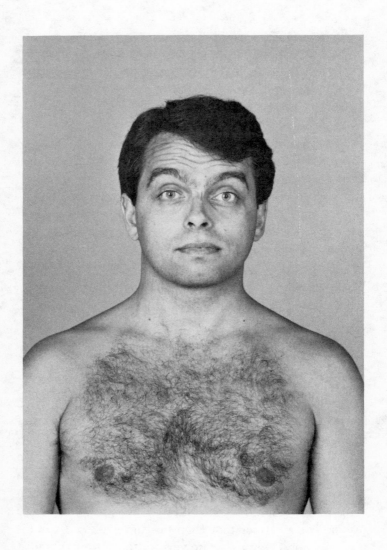

FOREHEAD TENSION / RELAXATION

FOREHEAD TENSION / RELAXATION

Technique: Sitting with your head, neck, and trunk erect, raise your eyebrows as if to push them into the hairline. Hold the tension for five seconds and then release. Do this three times. Close your eyes for thirty seconds upon completion of the exercise.

Points to Notice: Be aware of how you pull the tension tighter and tighter on the forehead, and how it travels across the scalp. Notice your eye movement, and when you release, be aware of the sensation that continues. For example, do you experience blood flow as pressure, colors, or sounds?

Purpose: This exercise puts you in the position of recognizing the sensation of tension in the forehead so that you can release it at other times of the day when the sensation comes forward.

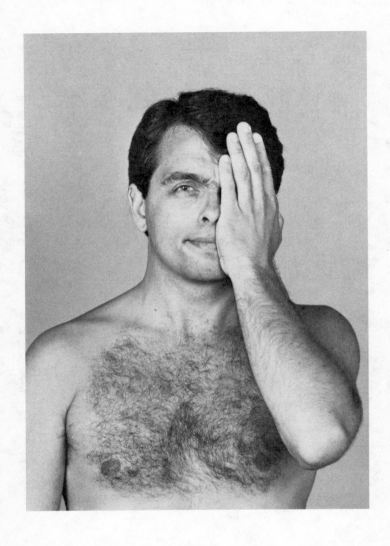

RIGHT / LEFT SIDE OF FACE TENSION / RELAXATION

RIGHT / LEFT SIDE OF FACE
TENSION / RELAXATION

Technique: Draw the muscles of the right side of your face into a state of tension in an extreme squint, while leaving the left side of your face free of the tension. If there is difficulty in doing so, place your left hand on the left side of your face to immobilize it so that the muscles can be found and isolated to bring the exercise into frution. Release. Then switch, and repeat the same on the other side. Do this exercise three times on each side of your face.

Points to Notice: During this exercise be aware of the sensation associated with tension on one side, and the absence of tension on the other side of your face. After completion, be aware of the experience in your face and notice whether or not it is symmetrical.

Purpose: As said earlier in this book, discrimination is very valuable in yoga therapy. This exercise is an opportunity to explore muscular discrimination. The request to move one side of the face and not the other requires fine muscular sensitivity. The intention here is to create a context for drawing distinctions, and to translate it with this discriminative faculty, into other areas.

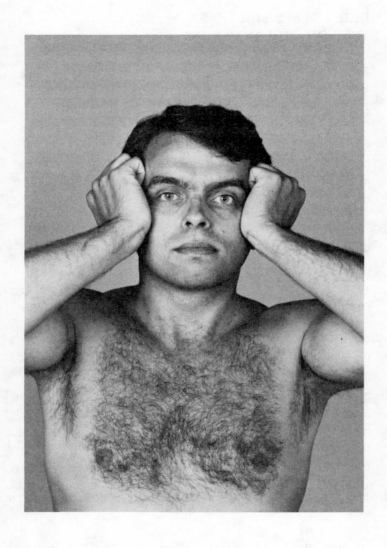

FOREHEAD / SINUS / FACE MASSAGE

FOREHEAD / SINUS / FACE MASSAGE

Technique: Place the heels of your hands to your forehead and begin to make gentle, slow, circular motions, massaging in turn the forehead, sinus area, temples, cheekbones, cheeks, jaw, and chin. Let go. Experience the facial muscles surrendering to your hands. Close your eyes and lower your hands.

Points to Notice: Be aware of the sensations that continue in your face after the massage is finished. Notice also the surrender of the facial tissue to the hands. Notice the sense of caress and kindness that the hands deliver to your face, experiencing being nice to yourself through the healing and relieving contact of the hands to the face.

Purpose: As awareness of the muscles of the face increase over the weeks, individual clients will become aware of tension as it begins to creep across their face, and will have a choice to employ the skills learned in therapy.

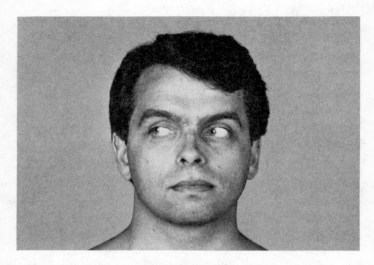

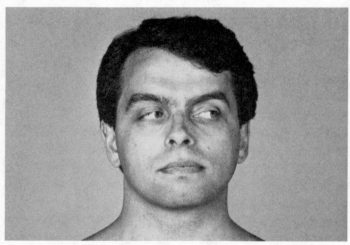

EYE EXERCISES

EYE EXERCISES

Technique: Starting with your eyes gazing straight ahead, turn your eyes sharply to the right without moving your head at all. Hold the tension for a short time, return to center. Relax. Repeat on the left side.

Bring your gaze up to the center between the eyebrows. Hold. Return to center and relax.

Take the gaze to the point where the nostrils meet the upper lip. Hold. Return to center. Relax.

Look up forty-five degrees to the right. Hold. Return to center, and relax.

Look down forty-five degrees to the left. Hold. Return to center, and relax.

Look up forty-five degrees to the left. Hold. Return to center, and relax.

Look down forty-five degrees to the right. Hold. Return to center and relax.

Rotate the eyes a full circle, going through each of the eight positions of the eyes on your way around. Rotate three times slowly in each direction. Close your eyes for a full sixty seconds.

Points to Notice: Be aware of the specific muscles involved in creating tension during this exercise. Each time you pause in the center, be sure you give yourself a few seconds to fully experience the relaxation. Notice the traveling of pressure across the skull. When your eyes rotate in a circle, be mindful that you do not skip any sections of the circle. There are tendencies to skip even full quadrants in the rotation. When you close your eyes, experience the sensations or images that will continue.

Purpose: I have found that many people carry tension in the muscles surrounding the eyes. Straining to see, or avoiding seeing will manifest around the eyes. This exercise will help to relieve some of the muscular tension in the eye area. Skipping sections of the eye during the rotation section may be associated with repressed material in the memory.

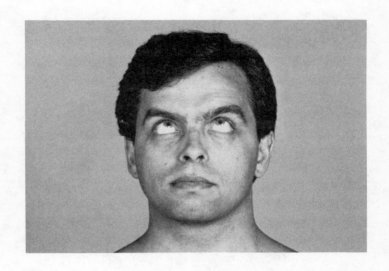

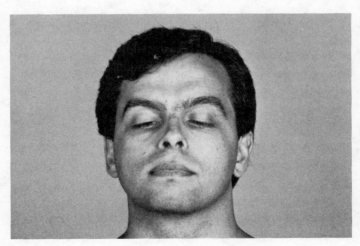

EYE EXERCISES

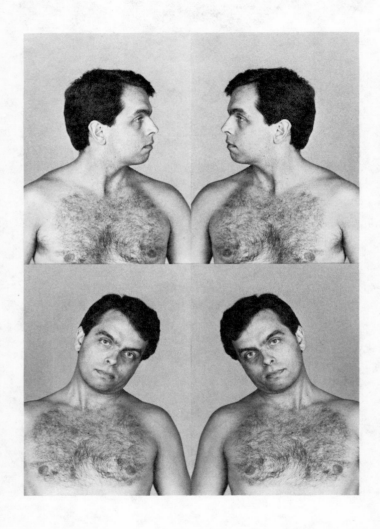

NECK EXERCISES

NECK EXERCISES

Technique: Sitting with your head, neck, and trunk erect, keep the torso facing forward throughout the exercise. On an exhalation, turn your head to the left as far as you can, as if looking over your left shoulder. On the inhalation return to the center, pause, and relax. On the exhalation, turn your head to the right as far as you can, as if looking over your right shoulder. On the inhalation return to the center, pause, and relax.

On the next exhalation, lean your head to the left as if touching the ear to the shoulder. On the inhalation, return to the center, pause, and relax. On an exhalation, lean your head to the right as if touching the ear to the shoulder. On the inhalation, return to the center, pause, and relax.

On the next exhalation bring your chin to your chest. Inhale as your bring your head up. On the exhalation, tilt your head back as far as you can. Inhale, and return to the center.

Lastly, on the exhalation, thrust your head forward as far as you can. Return to the center with the inhalation. On the exhalation tuck the chin back and in. Return to the center with the inhalation.

Close your eyes and reflect on the sensations for thirty seconds.

Points to Notice: During this exercise be aware of the pull of each muscle group and what constitutes the limit of your ability, be it tightness of muscle, pain, nausea, fear, defocusing of the eyes, etc. At the end of the exercise be aware of the wealth of information that continues even though you have completed the exercise.

Purpose: A large portion of the population stores stress in the neck and shoulder area. The purpose of this exercise is to relieve stress in those places. The promotion of blood circulation in this exercise can relieve headaches caused by pressure in the head. The learned sensitivity to the neuro-muscular functions of the shoulders and the neck will in the future alert the client that stress responses are building, allowing him to first, stop suppressive behavior, second, acknowledge that the current situation is stressful, and third, be in the position to employ additional options given in the therapeutic environment.

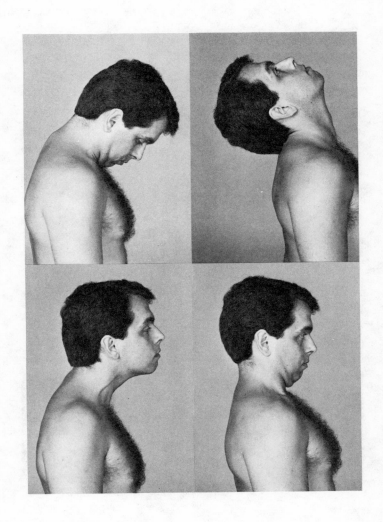

NECK EXERCISES

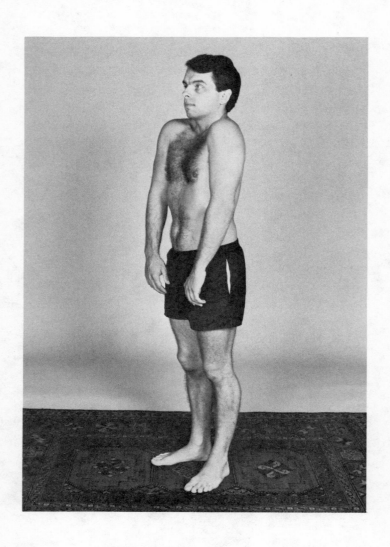

SHOULDER EXERCISES

SHOULDER EXERCISES

Technique: Slowly raise your right shoulder up to your right ear, and then let it drop. Repeat the same with the left shoulder. Do this three times.

Rotate the right shoulder in a complete circle: as far forward as you can, as far up as you can, as far back as you can, and as far down as you can. Make as large a circle as possible three times. Then reverse the direction and repeat three times. Follow the same procedure for the left shoulder.

Next perform all three exercises with both shoulders simultaneously. Coordinate your breath with the movement of your body. Inhale when the chest is opened and exhale when the back is opened. Do this three times in each direction.

Close your eyes at the end of the exercises.

Points to Notice: Be aware of the specific muscle groups and their flexibility or lack of it. Observe if you skip quadrants of the circle in the performance of the exercise. This will let you know if defenses are based in the chest or the back. Also notice if there is any difficulty in coordinating the breath with the motor skills. At the end of the exercise be aware of your personal pool of experiences and notice if there are emotional shifts.

Purpose: Many emotions are stored in the chest and back. This exercise may bring forward issues associated with vulnerability and personal expressiveness.

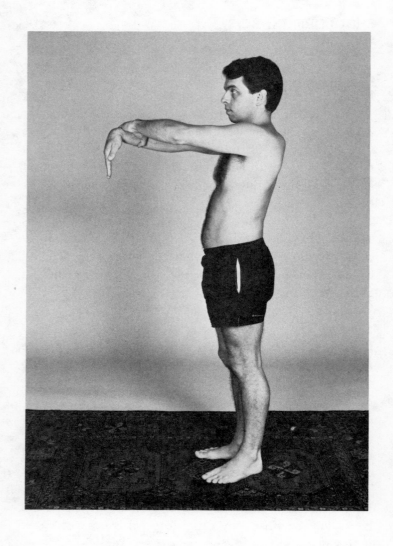

WRIST EXERCISE

WRIST EXERCISE

Technique: Hold your arms out straight in front of you parallel to the floor with the fingers extended and palms down. Rotate the hands at the wrist in as large a circle as possible. The forearms are not to be involved at all in this practice. Do first one wrist and then the other. Then do both wrists at the same time. Lower your arms to your side.

If there is any difficulty in isolating hand mobility from forearm immobility hold the forearm firmly with the other hand so that you can easily experience this isolation. At some point, the system will unconsciously learn to isolate.

Points to Notice: Be aware of sensations in the hands and fingers, and notice if there is any corresponding sensation in any area of the body.

Purpose: The aim of this exercise is to restructure the individual's sense of connectedness to his body by giving a task that requires concentration. This is one way to begin to create an experience of "groundedness" with the body—being present and aware inside of one's own body rather than disassociating out of defensiveness.

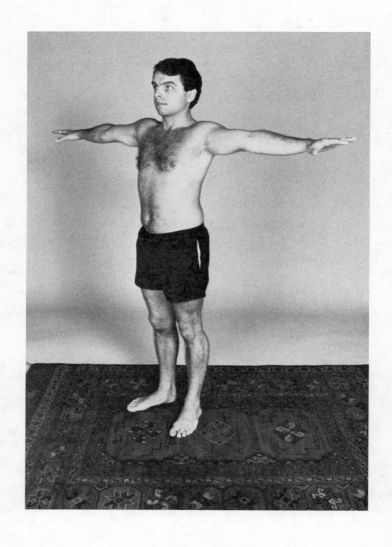

HORIZONTAL STRETCH

HORIZONTAL AND VERTICAL STRETCHES

Technique for Horizontal Stretch: Keeping both feet flat on the floor, extend both of your arms out to the sides as far as you can. Extend further at the shoulders, stretching the upper arms out further still. Open your elbows by extending them out, and make the forearms extend as if they were getting longer. Pull out at the wrist, extending the palms of your hands, the fingers, and the finger joints longer and longer still. Stretch out at the finger tips. Then release and let the arms drop by the sides. Close your eyes and reflect.

Technique for Vertical Stretch: Keeping the feet flat on the floor the entire duration of this exercise, raise the arms over the head, and stretch the body up at the ankles. Stretching up further through the calf muscles and the knees, pull the thighs up. Bring yourself up at the hips, extending the waist up further, and open up your rib cage. Stretching the shoulders up to the ears, stretch up the head and neck. Now the upper arms get longer, elbows reaching, forearms getting longer, the wrists pulling, finger joints getting longer, the finger tips stretching further still. Then let your arms down by your sides and close your eyes.

Points to Notice: Be aware of your ability to isolate your awareness to each segment of the body during both the horizontal and vertical stretches. When you release and close your eyes, be aware of the ongoing sensations most assuredly moving through your body.

Purpose: This is an opportunity to release general

tension in the muscles. In a group setting, one will typically find people sighing, while a look of release moves across their faces. Some will not be able to drop their arms at their sides, but will instead lower their arms to their sides. I take this as a sign of one's inability to "let go." In working with behavioral problem adolescents, I use this as a bias to observe whether they have the ability to psychologically "reach out" or reach "up and beyond" themselves.

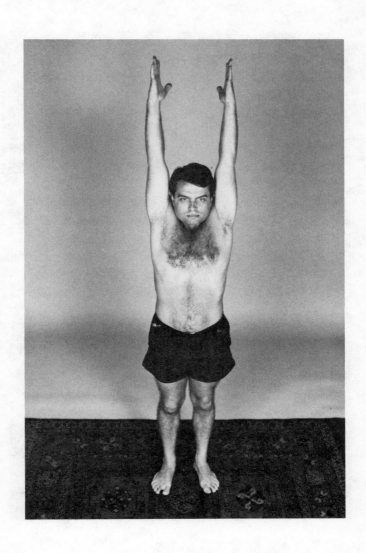

VERTICAL STRETCH

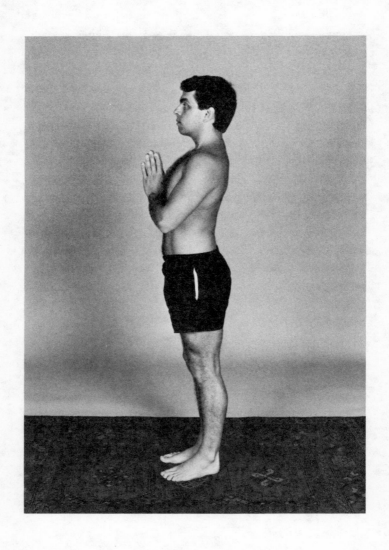

SOLAR SALUTATION / POSITION 1

SOLAR SALUTATION

Technique: Standing with your head, neck, and trunk erect, follow the next twelve positions.

Position 1: Plant both feet firmly on the ground, placing your hands, palms together, in front of your chest.

Position 2: Raise your arms over your head, palms facing each other a shoulder's width apart, and your weight over the instep. Inhale, and as you do so, arch back by first assuming the extended spine position of the vertical stretch. In arching back, however, do not collapse the spine, but require the front of your body to stretch over the extended spine.

Position 3: Leading with your chest, bend forward, exhaling as you do so, and keeping the arms and head raised. Flatten the back and roll the buttocks toward the ceiling in order to stretch the hamstrings, buttocks, and lower back. Place the hands to the knee, shin, ankle, foot, or the foor on either side of the feet, depending upon your capacity.

Position 4: Place one foot straight back, the ball of the foot to the floor. Bend the other leg at the knee so that the bent leg has its shin perpendicular to the floor and the top of the thigh parallel to the floor. This will require that your hips be down. Inhale while doing this position.

Position 5: While exhaling, bring the bent leg back to the other so that both feet are together. This will bring

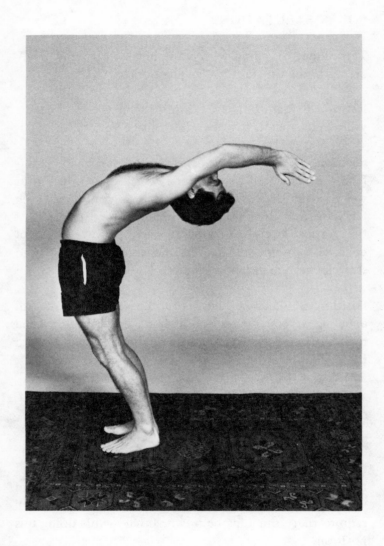

SOLAR SALUTATION / POSITION 2

both hands and both feet to the floor in a quadruped position. Roll your buttocks to the ceiling, pressing your heels toward the floor while stretching the lower back and hamstring muscles. Do not walk the hands and feet toward each other.

Position 6: Continuing to exhale from Position 5, bring your toes, knees, chest, and forehead into contact with the floor.

Position 7: With the inhalation, lower the body to the floor, point the toes, raise the head and chest off the floor, and slowly straighten the arms, tucking the pelvis so as to give support to the lower back. Roll the shoulders back to open the chest, and push the head back to complete the pose.

Position 8: With the exhalation, lower the body to the floor again. Bring the balls of the feet back underneath the feet and pike up, repeating Position 5, and remembering to roll the buttocks to the ceiling.

Position 9: With the inhalation, lunge forward with the foot that was put straight back first in Position 4, duplicating Position 4. The tip of this foot is to come into straight alignment with the fingertips.

Position 10: With the exhalation, bring both feet forward between your hands and straighten your legs. This will then be the same as Position 3.

Position 11:   Ensuring that your weight is evenly distributed on your feet, right to left and back to

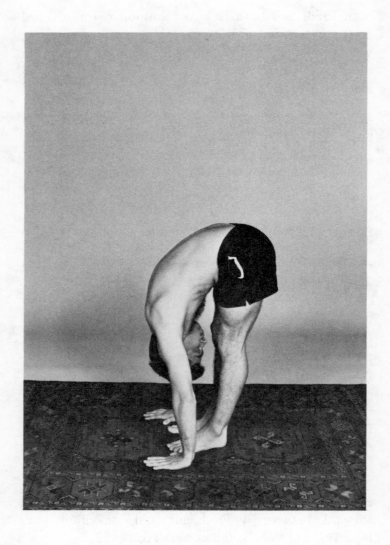

SOLAR SALUTATION / POSITION 3

front, inhale and raise your hands, head, and shoulders in order to flatten the spine. (Caution: watch out for dizziness.) Keeping the spine flattened and the arms extended, come to an erect position, lengthening the spine again as in the vertical stretch. Arch back to your capacity, stretching the front of the body over the spine.

Position 12: With the exhalation, come back to an erect position, hands clasped in front of the chest as in Position 1.

This exercise should be done from three to six times. In the beginning you may not want to coordinate the movement of the body and the breath, until you no longer need to read the instructions.

Points to Notice: Be aware of specific muscle groups involved in the performance of each position of the posture. Notice your breath rhythms, balance, strength or lack of strength, flexibility or its lack. Be aware of your emotions, such as panic, fear, pleasure, nervousness, to name a few.

Purpose: This posture is used as an opportunity to experience the recovery mechanism in action. The return to a state of homeostasis is an unconscious function. Here, however, after guiding the organism to excel, you have the opportunity to learn physical recovery procedure coupled with the intention of self-awareness. I have found that when a human being involves himself in any environment repeatedly, he will eventually learn the system and gain control over it. The control in this

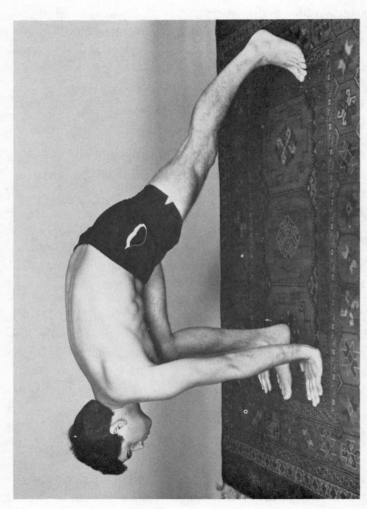

SOLAR SALUTATION / POSITION 4

case is learning how to let the recovery mechanism operate, thus allowing for intercession—speeding up of the recovery process. This intercession can take place because through self-observation the human being will be able to make finer distinctions inside the system.

I also use the Solar Salutation to observe how familiar a client is with his body. I particularly observe his balance or lack thereof. If there is unawareness of a body part, there will be a tendency to lose balance with one of the positions. I look for unevenness of strength. For example, weak arms may be a metaphor showing that one's arms are incapable of supporting him in the world. How does he handle being taxed for an outcome? Does he quit? Get challenged? Become defiant? Under what circumstances and by what criteria does he determine what his limits are? I usually voice these questions for the group to ponder.

This exercise is a good overall toner, and has an aerobic feature to it which is very valuable for a sedentary lifestyle.

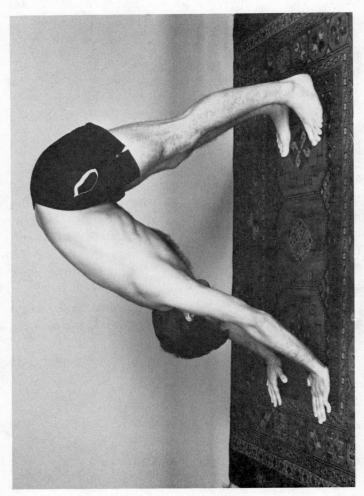

SOLAR SALUTATION / POSITION 5

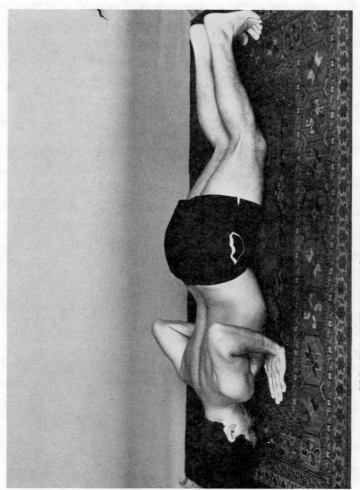

SOLAR SALUTATION / POSITION 6

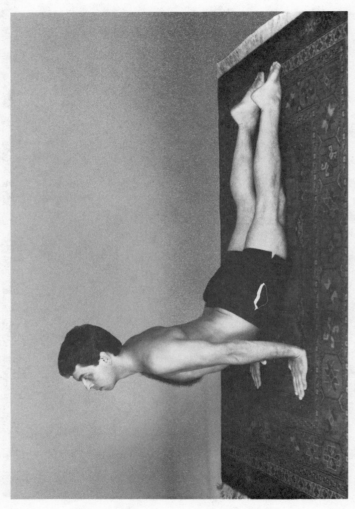

SOLAR SALUTATION / POSITION 7

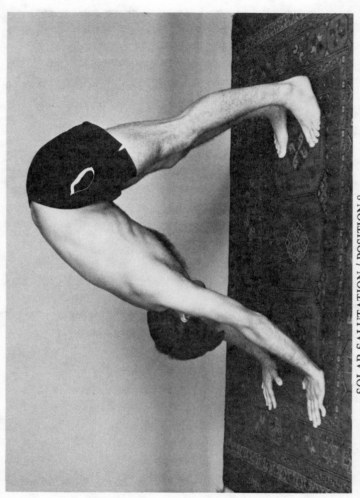

SOLAR SALUTATION / POSITION 8

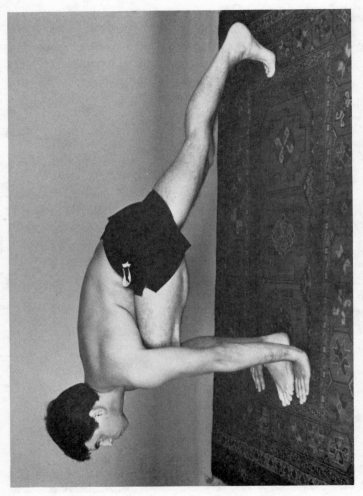

SOLAR SALUTATION / POSITION 9

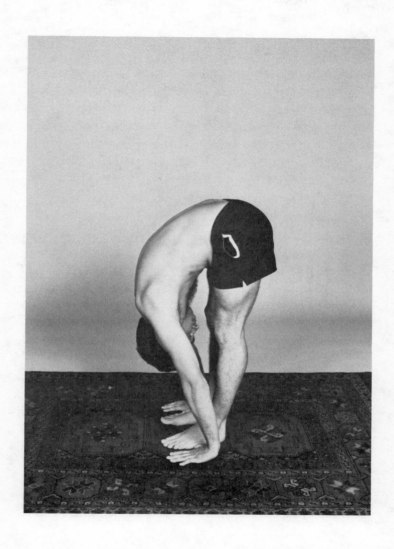

SOLAR SALUTATION / POSITION 10

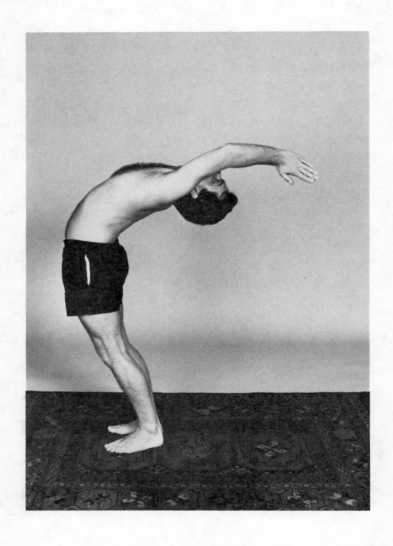

SOLAR SALUTATION / POSITION 11

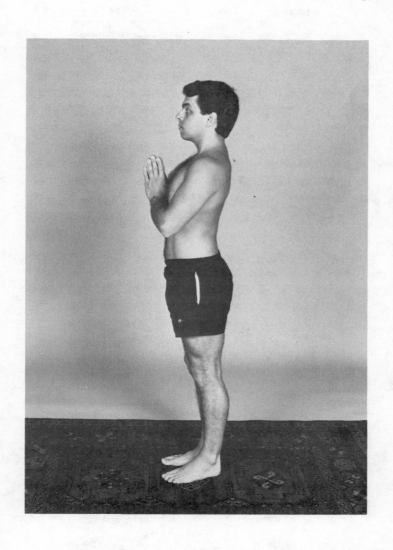

SOLAR SALUTATION / POSITION 12

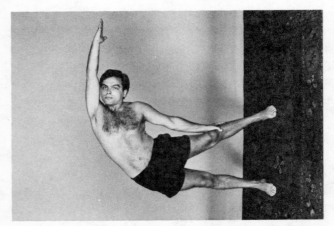

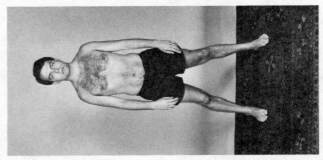

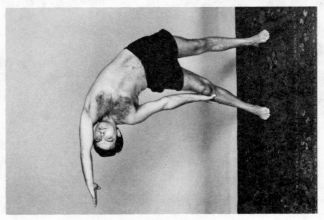

SIDE BEND

SIDE BEND

Technique: Inhale, exhale, and spread your feet about three feet apart. Extend your right hand down your right leg and lean your torso to the right side directly over your hipbone. Keep your ankle, knee, hip, rib cage, shoulder, and head in the same line as when standing. This means you will not extend your hips to the back or the front, but move straight over to the right side. To intensify this stretch, bring the left straightened arm to the left ear. Breathe deeply. Return to center. Repeat the same movement on the left side. Breathe deeply so as to stretch the intercostal muscles (muscles between the ribs).

Points to Notice: Be aware of the pull on the extended side of your rib cage. As a caution note that it is very easy to overextend in this pose.

Purpose: This posture is useful to release levels of stored tension in the intercostal muscles accumulated during the retention or diminishment of breath in stressful periods. The opening of the rib cage in this and other poses will allow the lungs to move more freely and easily.

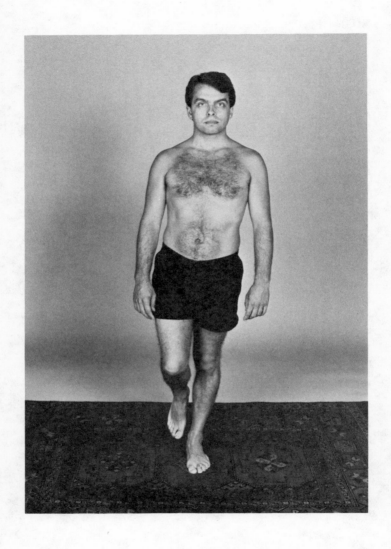

BALANCE ON ONE FOOT

BALANCE ON ONE FOOT

Technique: Raise the right foot off the floor, and balance on the left foot. Switch sides and do the same.

With both feet on the floor, come up onto the balls of the feet and balance. Lower.

Raise the right foot, come up on the ball of the left foot and balance. Lower and do the same thing on the other side.

Pause and reflect.

Points to Notice: Be aware of your balance, and the internal dialogue that takes place while doing the pose. Notice if it is easier to balance on one side of the body rather than the other.

Purpose: I use this posture as an indicator of how well a client orients himself in the world through his stability in gravity, and use improvements in the pose as an indicator of where he is with himself and his therapy. I notice that the reasons articulated in internal dialogue for falling out of the pose are of the same context as reasons for other instabilities in life. This pose is a wonderful non-threatening way to access this information.

There is oftentimes a right/left, top/bottom or criss-cross split in a person's physical development. This asymmetry in the body is a reflection of other levels of uneven or conflicting inner developmental patterns. If you notice a person consistently having issues associated with one side of the body or another, you might consider targeting your coaching to bring about a reconciliation within the individual. This asymmetry may manifest in bruising one side of the body more than another, total ineptness of one side of the body, obvious disparity between the two sides in growth, or in this case, one-sided balance.

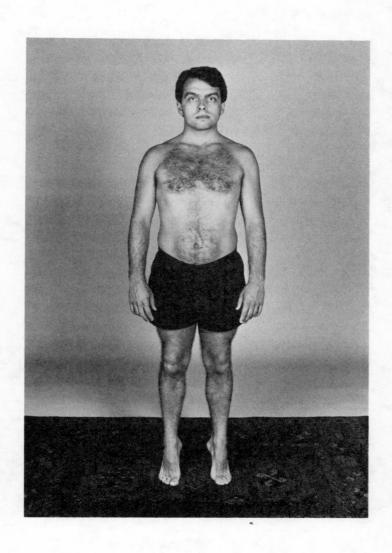

BALANCE ON ONE FOOT

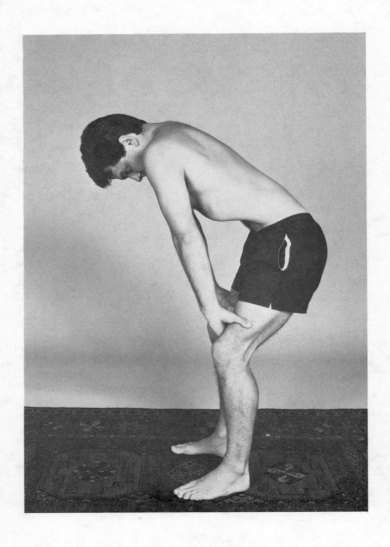

ABDOMINAL LIFT

ABDOMINAL LIFT

Caution: If there are difficulties with the heart, severe asthma, or epilepsy, do not do this practice unless you consult a physician. It also should not be done during pregnancy.

Technique: With both feet squarely on the floor, bend both legs slightly at the knees. Rest each hand on its respective thigh. Exhale and empty your lungs completely. With the lungs empty, contract the abdominal muscles toward your back as far as possible. Press your chin against your throat and contract the pelvic floor, especially closing the anal sphincters.

Hold the muscles contracted until you feel the urge to inhale. Release the abdominal muscles, and let the breath rush back into the lungs through the nostrils. Catch your breath, and do the exercise a second and a third time. Pause and reflect upon whatever information passes through your organism.

Points to Notice: Be aware of the anal sphincters, ensuring that they are pulled up. Notice the internal dialogue that is associated with deciding when to resume breathing.

Purpose: This exercise will aid in reconnecting and restimulating suppressed issues in those who disassociate from emotions in the abdominal and pelvic regions (that is, power, fear, sex), by locking their muscles or internal organs in this area. It is also helpful for those who suppress emotions as a defensive posture.

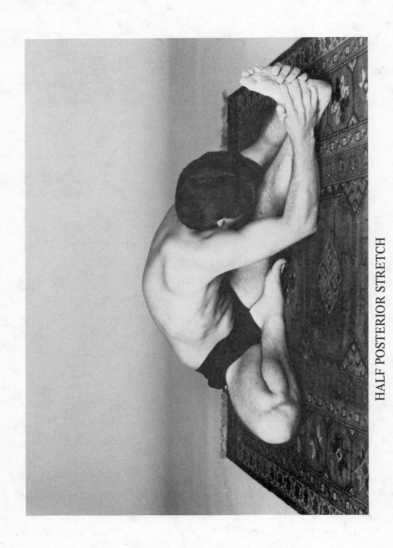

HALF POSTERIOR STRETCH

HALF POSTERIOR STRETCH

Technique: Sitting on the floor, extend both legs out in front of you, flexing the feet by extending the heel as far away from you as possible. Bend the right leg at the knee, drawing the heel in toward the perineum while pressing the knee down toward the floor.

While inhaling, raise the arms over the head. Stretch up, and with the exhalation, lean forward over your straightened leg and grasp your toes, knees, calves, or your foot, depending upon your capacity. Your intention is to take the abdomen down toward the thigh, the chest toward the knee, and the top of the head toward the foot. Keeping the left leg straight, press the back of the left knee toward the floor. Depending upon your flexibility, continue to press the bent right knee toward the floor so as to open the tendons at the groin. Make sure that the shoulders are level as there is a tendency for the shoulder on the right to be lower. By pressing the left shoulder down you will increase the pull across the entire body. Hold for thirty seconds in the beginning and increase the time slowly.

Release, massaging whichever portion of the body may need loosening. Then do the same on the other side of the body.

Points to Notice: Ensure that the abdomen moves toward the thigh. This will stretch the lower back, buttocks, and hamstring muscles.

Purpose: Rotating the pelvis open on one side and then on the other can help to ease some of the tension stored in the hip joints. Posterior stretch benefits also apply.

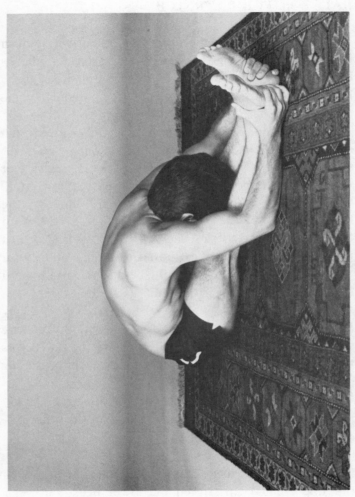

POSTERIOR STRETCH

POSTERIOR STRETCH

Technique: While sitting on the floor, extend both legs straight out in front of you, flexing the foot by extending the heel as far away from you as possible and pressing the back of the knees toward the floor. Sitting with the head, neck, and trunk erect, exhale. During the inhalation, raise the arms over the head, stretching the body up. As you exhale, lean forward, keeping the back flat and rotating the buttocks back. Reach forward and grasp as far down your legs as you can, using the leverage to stretch your body even further.

Points to Notice: Be aware of where you experience the resistance to the posture in your body. It may feel as if your entire body is resisting, but find what parts specifically are central to the resistance. Once you locate the specific area of the resistance, define its parameters: How far up does it extend? How far down? How far to each side? How deep? Now mentally enter the center of the resistance with a calm, relaxed attitude.

To bring ease some students imagine water. Some find it helpful to imagine the tension going out with the exhalation, and flooding the tense area with an experience of ease or light on the inhalation. Others have found that imagining or inducing a sound vibration in the area of resistance will release the tightness. After you have done this, you may notice that the tension has decreased to a noticeable degree. If so, pursue the posture by lowering the torso further still.

Purpose: I have an interesting proposition for you to explore. Consider the possibility that the back side of the body may be associated with deep, unconscious armoring, and the front part of the body associated with conscious and more superficial levels of unconscious armoring. Remember that the front of the body of a biped leads into the world, vulnerable and accessible; whereas a quadruped leads with the head only as vulnerable. I have noticed in my study of body language that unconscious blocks tend to manifest in the back of the body. This posture addresses, through a stretch of the lower back, issues associated with suppression of sexual expression and a personal sense of power in the sense of directing one's own life. I have also found that these two are very closely related.

CRADLING THE LEGS

Technique: Sitting with the head, neck, and trunk erect, raise the left leg, bend it at the knee, and cradle the left foot in the bend of the right elbow. Cradle the left thigh in the bend of the left elbow, and join the fingers of the hands together. This requires some flexibility. Stretch your back as much as you can, and gently rock the cradled leg in your arms.

Then release the thigh with the left arm, putting both arms around the left foot and drawing the foot into or towards the pelvis. Raise the foot to the navel, then the chest, then toward the face. Lower the foot to the floor and go through the same procedure with the right leg.

Points to Notice: Be aware of how you define your limits. Be sure to keep the back as straight as possible. Notice which part of your body is offering the resistance, as this may change as you progress. In the beginning, for instance, you may experience the major resistance in the back of your thigh. Later on, as the thigh loosens, the resistance may shift to the buttocks or lower back. Remember to breathe throughout the exercise.

Purpose: This posture again works on the back side of the body and targets somewhat similar to the posterior stretch.

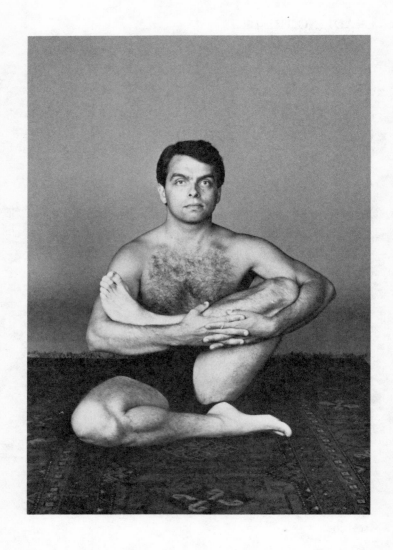

CRADLING THE LEGS

LATERAL TWISTING OF THE SPINE
IN THE EASY CROSS-LEGGED POSTURE

Technique: Sitting with the head, neck, and trunk erect, and legs in a crossed position, inhale, then exhale and place the right hand on the floor behind you. Twist the torso to the right, completing the twist by looking over the right shoulder. Keeping the spine erect, place the left hand at the right knee. Using the left hand as leverage, pull the left shoulder across the body, twisting the torso around even further. Hold for thirty seconds, keeping the spine erect, the chest open, and the pelvis facing front. Exhale and inhale, expanding the chest as you do so.

Release, return to center, and go through the same process on the left side by putting the left hand on the floor behind you.

Points to Notice: Be sure that you continue to breathe, and that the chest opens around the erect spine. Ensure that the twist is completed by turning your head around as far as you can. Upon completion close your eyes and notice your breathing, images, and internal dialogue. Also note if there is an experience of heat in the lower back and chest.

Purpose: The motion of the body in this posture is somewhat similar to wringing a towel. It expands the chest and stimulates blood circulation in the muscles of the back at the spine. It also assists in removing tension in the muscles of the back so those suffering from lower back pain can be helped by its use.

I notice that some clients have difficulty in twisting

backwards, especially when turning the head and neck to the rear to complete the twist. In my own belief system and history I explore whether or not this person has issues in his past that he does not want to look upon. This may sound a little far-fetched for those who are pragmatically minded, but my experience has shown me that this is a valuable bias.

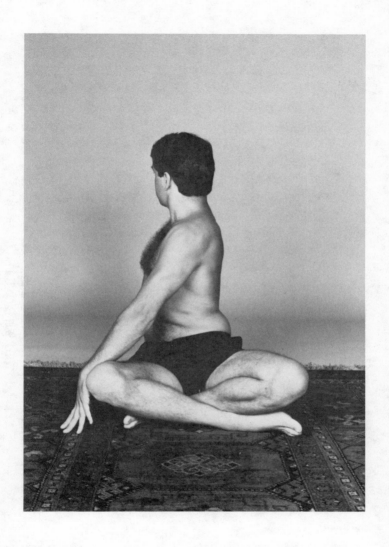

LATERAL TWISTING OF THE SPINE
IN THE EASY CROSS-LEGGED POSTURE

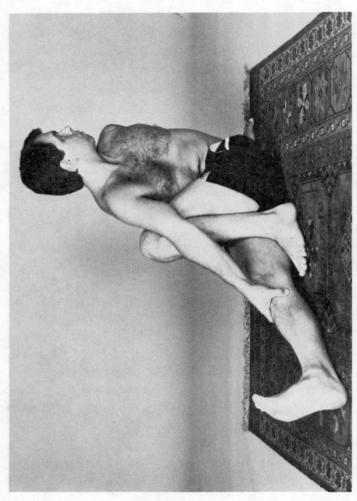

SPINAL TWIST WITH ONE LEG STRAIGHT

SPINAL TWIST WITH ONE LEG STRAIGHT

Technique: Sitting with the head, neck, and trunk erect, extend your right leg straight out in front of you. Bending your left leg at the knee, draw the heel to the perineum and the thigh to the chest as you inhale. Exhale and twist to the left, placing the left hand on the floor behind you. Twist the torso to the left as far as you can, crossing the right arm and shoulder over the left leg. Place the right upper arm against the outside of the left leg. Eventually the left knee should be behind the right shoulder. Exhale and inhale deeply to open your chest. Using the right arm or shoulder as leverage, exhale and push around even further, finishing the twist by turning the head as if to look over the left shoulder. Hold the spine erect and open the chest as much as you can.

Release. Return to center and go through the same process on the right side by trading leg positions and twisting to the right.

Points to Notice: Be aware of all the recommendations in the previous cross-legged twist, and make sure your legs are in the correct places. You may find that exhaling and contracting the abdominal muscles will allow you to twist even further. Be sure to breathe during the posture.

Purpose: The purpose of this pose is the same as that of the simple twist. It differs only in the sense that it is more intense in the requirements that it places upon the body. I say this because the application of this posture and its many variations in more advanced

hatha yoga training are designed to impact the energy
of the digestive and eliminative systems, in addition to
aiding spinal flexibility. These particular issues, however, are not within the scope of this book.

In terms of spinal flexibility, I have noticed in my
observation of people, that as one progresses in age,
those whose spines are erect seem to be more vital.
Those who are bent over are apparently not in a state
of full human ease and vitality and usually have some
walking aid.

CROCODILE

Technique: Lie down on the floor on the front of your body. Fold your arms by placing your hands on your upper arms, and rest your forehead on your forearms. Spread your feet apart a distance that you personally find comfortable.

Breathe deeply.

Points to Notice: Be aware of your breath. You can do this by experiencing any of the various forms of the breath, for example, listening to the sound of the breath in the hollow created in your arms; feeling its moisture on your face; noticing the rise and fall of your back; or the pressure of your abdominal wall against the floor.

Purpose: This posture is used for relaxation. The use of this posture will generate a deep feeling of relaxation. This is caused in part by the weight being put upon the breathing mechanism. It slows the breath down and tends to move the mechanics of the breath into the abdominal region.

This posture will quickly bring back into a state of relaxing ease anyone who is suffering an anxiety attack. Anyone who is hypertense, however, may find this, and other relaxation postures, anxiety-producing, because the relaxation response that begins to move through the nervous system causes him to begin to loosen some of his defense mechanisms. This will allow the system to be excited again with memories of the old behavior, and the individual may report that he feels like crawling out of his skin, or getting up and running out of the room.

In such a case, I would recommend the tension/relaxation exercises from the next chapter and/or the breathing techniques described in chapter eleven.

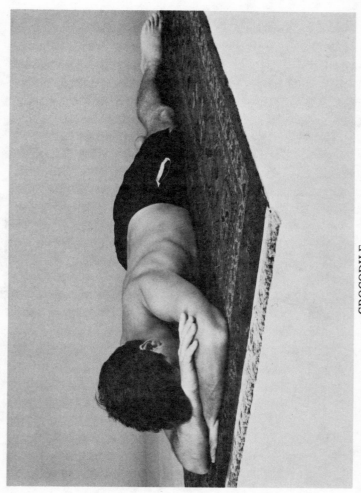

CROCODILE

212

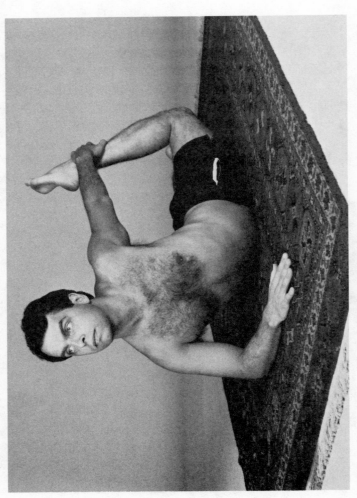

HALF BOW POSE

HALF BOW POSE

Technique: Lying face down with your arms in the same position as in the crocodile pose, bend the right leg at the knee. Reach back with your right hand and grasp the right ankle. Raise your head, and while exhaling, push back with the right leg, pulling against the right hand. This will arch your right thigh and your chest off the floor. For those of you who are too stiff to reach your ankle with your hand, you can use a tie, looping it around your ankle, grasping it with your right hand, and then pulling.

Exhale, release, and go through the same process on the other side. If you experience a need for your lower back to be stretched at the completion of the posture, go to the child's pose.

Points to Notice: Be aware of the pressure at your knee. Some may feel excessive strain in that area. Notice where you experience lack of flexibility in your body. Is it in your shoulder? Chest? Thigh? Back? Notice if one side of the body is more open than the other, as this can be used as data for therapeutic outcomes. Continue to breathe during the exercise.

Purpose: The purpose of this pose is to open the front of the body. The natural tightening defensive reflex of one's biped vulnerability will translate into armoring in the system if not loosened when one has matured beyond its need. Like the full bow pose, this posture stretches the front of the body over the back like a rack. It looks as if you are bending the back in these postures, yet a main requirement is that the front loosen to stretch over the back. Thus to bring about a more expansive opening of the front of the body it is very important to lengthen the spine as you arch back, as in the solar salutation.

Knee difficulties are associated with ego strength, in the sense of one's inner work and struggle with oneself. If a client's knees are weak, I ask if he is experiencing being vanquished by another. A colleague of mine, Dr. Vijayendra Pratap, did extensive work on the psychological implications of the bending of the knees. He noted that the kees were bent in acts of surrender: prayer, paying obeisance before a recognized power, initiation, submission, pleading. The terms "weak kneed" or "trembling knees" demonstrate an unconscious collective understanding of the psychological significance of this area of the body.

Ego strength issues associated with the lower back, on the other hand, are related to ego strength in regards to confidence with the sexual center, needs fulfillment, and feelings of oppression (as if someone had his foot in your back).

FULL BOW

Technique: Lying face down, bend both of your legs at the knees. Reach back with both hands and grasp each respective ankle. You may find that spreading the knees makes performance of this posture easier; as you become more adept the knees can be brought closer together.

Exhale and raise first your head and then your chest. Then push against the hands with the legs. Hold your head erect. Press the sternum forward so as to open the chest, and push the soles of the feet up as you press the legs against the hands. This will stretch the shoulders and chest open even more. Exhale and inhale.

Exhale and release. When you reach the floor, go to the child's pose if you experience that your lower back needs to be stretched.

Points to Notice: Be aware of how the breath expands your rib cage. For those of you who find their pelvic bones pressing against the floor, causing discomfort, put a folded blanket between the pelvis and the floor for cushioning. Again, a tie or rope may be used to pull the feet to the hands for those who do not have adequate flexibility. Notice if one side of your body is more flexible than the other, and also which side of the body fatigues before the other. This can be used as data for therapeutic intervention.

Purpose: As stated in the half pow bose, this posture opens the chest horizontally, and stretches vertically through the body. It also strengthens the breathing mechanism much like the crocodile pose, because one is resting on the abdomen (and in some cases the diaphragm), which requires lifting part of the body weight with each breath.

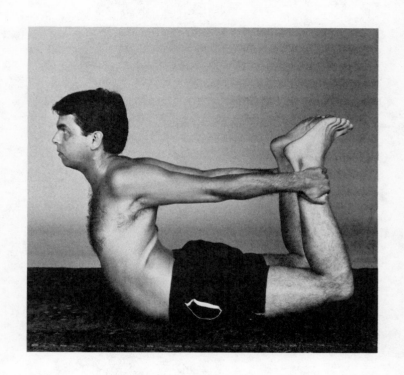

FULL BOW

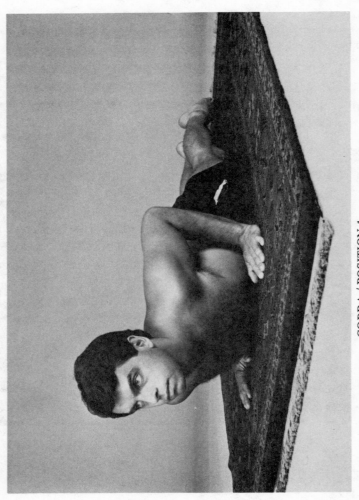

COBRA / POSITION 1

COBRA

Technique: Lie on the floor face down, legs together, toes pointed, hands under the shoulders, fingertips pointing straight ahead aligned with the shoulders, elbows close to the body. Exhale. You can use four following positions in this pose.

Position 1: Raise the head and chest without using the hands and arms. Tucking the pelvis and tightening the buttocks, come up as high as you can. Roll the shoulders back and stretch your throat and head up. Extend your spine, pulling the front of your body through your chest.

Position 2: Pressing your hands to the floor and stretching the body, come up further to the point where the navel remains on the floor, keeping your buttocks and lower back firm in order to keep the lower back protected. Roll your shoulders back, opening your chest as if you were to pop your buttons. The head goes back and you pull through the body.

Position 3: Keeping the toes pointed, press the hands against the floor. Continue up so that now the pelvis remains on the floor. Keep the back firm and roll the shoulders even further, stretching open through the front of the body.

Position 4: Pushing against the floor, straighten the arms completely so that the body will be hanging between the shoulders and thighs. Be sure to keep the pelvis tucked so as to protect the lower back.

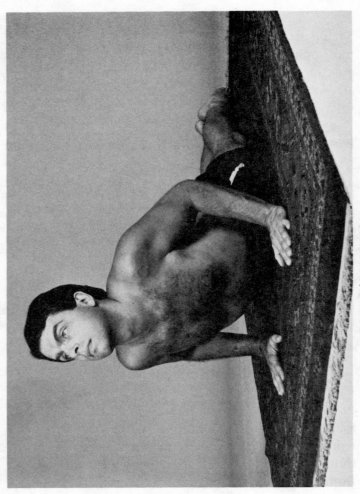

COBRA / POSITION 2

To release from all positions, press the front of the body, on the exhalation, slowly to the floor and lengthen the spine one vertebra at a time as you lower. When you reach the floor, if you experience that your lower back needs to be stretched, go to the child's pose.

Points to Notice: Be aware of your lower back through the entire process. Keep your feet together, pelvis tucked. Be sure to expand your chest during this exercise. Notice the spine and attempt to elongate it as you also stretch the front of the body.

Purpose: This pose is another used to open the front of the body and create flexibility in the spine. The different positions allow you to focus more specifically on portions of the front and back of the body with less physical effort. The stimulation of the muscles of the back promotes blood circulation to the back. This provides great benefit in keeping the back flexible during aging.

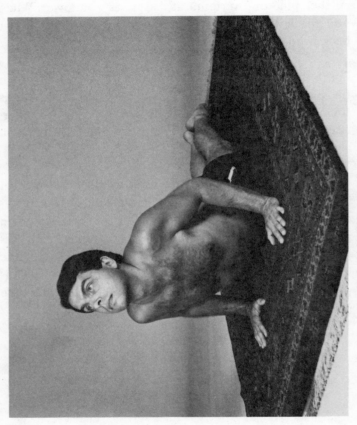

COBRA / POSITION 3

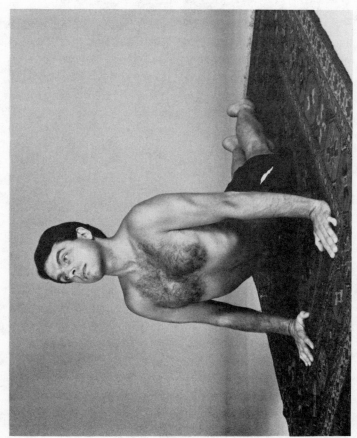

COBRA / POSITION 4

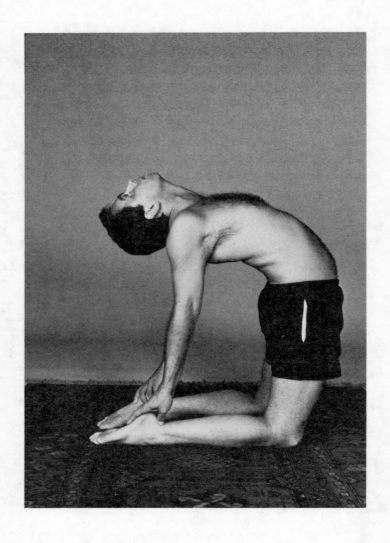

CAMEL

CAMEL

Technique: This posture can be done from two positions. Explore and find out which one suits you.

Position 1: Kneel with your knees spread apart the width of your hips. As you progress in this pose you will bring your knees toward each other. Sit to your heels and place your hands on your heels. Exhale and push the pelvis forward, raising the buttocks off the heels. Tuck your pelvis so as to support the lower back.

Position 2: Kneel, and while standing on your knees, exhale and arch back so that the hands will rest upon the feet. Grasp the heels and tuck the pelvis forward.

The next step applies to both positions. Tuck the pelvis forward in order to support the lower back. Press the front of the thighs forward, and roll the shoulders back, pressing the sternum towards the ceiling. Press the spine forward as if you were going to push the spine through the center of the chest. Let the head hang back and continue to press the pelvis and thighs further forward still. Exhale and inhale deeply to open the chest.

When you release, exhale, and either return to Position 1 by sitting to your heels, or return to Position 2. Then go to the child's pose.

Points to Notice: Be aware that you continue to keep the lower back strong. Press the chest to greater expansiveness. Breathe deeply. The knees should be watched in this pose to make sure you stay within the bounds of their capacity. Notice which portion of your body offers the resistance and what kinds of thoughts are stimulated while doing this pose.

Purpose: This posture has the same look as the bow, but in its performance you will find it stimulates different attitudes. Flexibility of the back does not necessarily mean that a person is psychologically flexible.

I have found that people who are extremely flexible in one direction, such as backwards, are sometimes not at all flexible in the opposite direction. This imbalance usually demonstrates itself in the personality. The extreme ability to bend back can translate as a "lack of spine" or an inability to stand up for oneself due to a lack of an inner core of personal strength.

CHILD'S POSE

Technique: Kneeling, sit to your heels either on top or between your heels, with your large toes touching at the tips. This can form a seat or cradle for your buttocks. Put your head to the floor at the knees, and at the beginning, if you like, stretch your back by extending your arms straight out in front of you, pulling all the way to the buttocks. Afterwards, release, put your arms back on the floor alongside your legs, and let your head remain on the floor.

Points to Notice: Be aware of your spine and the pull of each vertebra as you stretch. Notice the rhythm of your breath, for as you hold the pose it may slow. If there is any difficulty in breathing, spread your knees and lie down between your thighs.

Purpose: This posture is used for a number of reasons. Physically it stretches the lower back after doing intense back-bending poses. I encourage my students to use it to relieve tightness in the lower back in the course of a class as they deem it necessary, whether or not it is assigned.

The psychological value of this pose is that it can create a sense of security since it is the fetal position. The entire front of the body is covered, and so all of the vulnerable parts are safe. This generates a sense of security for the practitioner. We stiffen or hide to protect that which is essential in shaping our development. It is not wrong to want to protect oneself; the key is only to realize when old defensive behaviors are inappropriate. There must be an opening up to a position where one is strong enough to be vulnerable. This is called maturity. The child's pose is an acknowledgement of fetal safety. Standing erect or arching backwards is taking a risk with that safety.

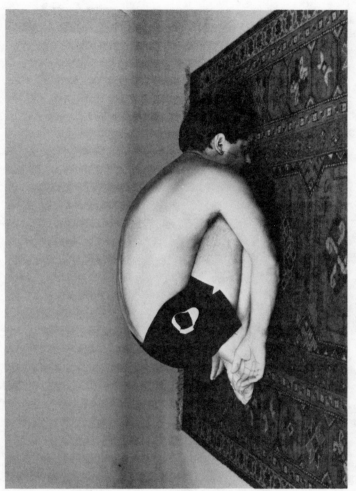

CHILD'S POSE

HALF LOCUST

HALF LOCUST

Technique: Lie face down, legs straight out behind you, arms to the floor alongside the body, and chin to the floor. Keep your legs straight and exhale. Raise one straightened leg in the air behind you. Keep your pelvis to the floor. There is a tendency to rotate the hip of the raised leg in the air, which changes the direction of the pull on the back. The palms can be turned down, or the hands can be made into a fist while the posture is being executed. Breathe normally. Exhale, and slowly lower to the floor. Do the same thing to the other side of the body.

Points to Notice: Be aware of the pull through the neck, upper back, lower back, buttocks, and back of the thighs. Notice if one side of the body is stronger than the other, and if one leg raises higher than the other. What point of your body stops you in the pose? Is it your hips? Thigh? Lower back?

Purpose: The purpose of this pose is to strengthen the back side of the body. I use it to assist clients in gaining ego strength at an unconscious level. There are many other ways to facilitate this, such as breathing and abdominal work.

In using this posture to collect data for therapeutic intervention, students can investigate whether their limits have been consistently delineated by the same part of the body. What criteria do they use to decide that they no longer have strength to hold the pose? I invite them to listen to their internal dialogue about this. As one forms reasons why he should stop, he may notice that he uses that line of logic to stop activity in other areas of his life as well, because he does not experience himself as having enough to go on. We all have our limits; this is to be expected. But these postures that tax our limits are a quick, safe way to approach our boundaries in order to evaluate our boundary-setting mechanism. We can then experiment with new criteria for boundary-setting in the postures, forming an apparently hypothetical paradigm for experimentation in other parts of our life, such as relationships, success, or failure.

FULL LOCUST

Technique: Lying face down, chin to the floor, arms lying by your side, place both straightened arms under your body. Make a fist with your balled hands on the floor under the pelvic girdle. Exhale and raise both straightened legs into the air as high as you can. Hold. Then gradually lower the legs to the floor.

Release. Do the pose a second and third time, and when you reach your capacity, sit to your heels and assume the child's pose.

Points to Notice: Be aware of the symmetry of your muscular strength as you raise into the pose. Are there emotions? In addition, see the points listed in the half locust pose.

Purpose: At this point in the postures you will be working with both hemispheres of the body in juxtaposition. This will allow you to notice which side is stronger and which side allows blood circulation (and thus energy), to flow more freely.

By observing people when they stand before you, you can notice that one side of the body is usually developed differently from the other. The tighter side will tend to be lower on the horizontal line because its contraction will overpower and pull the weaker side. This will cause resulting adjustments in other parts of the body. You may notice one eye lower than the other, one breast lower than the other, the head tilted more to one side than to the other.

My therapeutic intention is to invite clients to resume expanding into the world. I acknowledge them for having developed the strategies they have as a context for the current evolution of their personality. I then let them know that it is now time to release their current barriers and venture forth into the world to create new interactions with it. They must now invent a new definition of themselves, and set new limits to be exceeded at a later time.

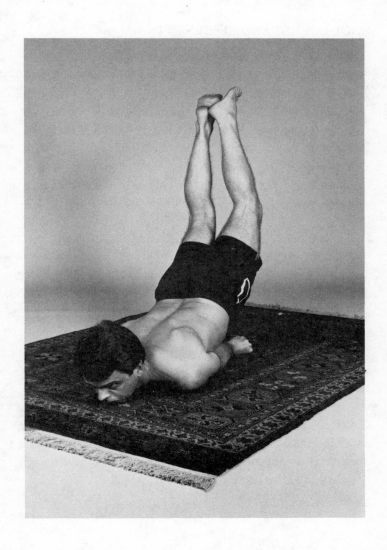

FULL LOCUST

SHOULDERSTAND SERIES

The shoulderstand series is a sequence developed from traditional postures. This series is composed of postures according to one's level of competency.

At the beginning level:
Shoulderstand, plow, lowering to the floor, bridge, and fish.

At the intermediate level:
Shoulderstand, plow, shoulderstand, bridge, shoulderstand, plow, lowering to the floor, and fish.

At the advanced level:
Shoulderstand, plow, shoulderstand, bridge, wheel, bridge, shoulderstand, plow, lower to the floor, fish.

I will describe each posture singularly. When you apply these postures, however, you can apply them in one of the above sequences. Do not be a slave to the sequence.

Caution: Always do the neck exercises before the shoulderstand or plow. The neck and shoulder muscles need warming up before they are required to go through the extreme stretching of these two poses.

SHOULDERSTAND

Caution: If you have disorders of high blood pressure or heart irregularities do not do this pose.

Technique: Lying on your back, legs straight, feet together, arms by your side, and palms down, raise both straightened legs into the air. Bend your knees, bring your knees to your forehead (this will take the pressure off your back), support your back with your hands, point your feet towards the ceiling, and raise your legs straight into the air. In the advanced application, instead of bending your knees, you would go to the plow, position your hands on your back, then raise your legs into the shoulderstand.

Strive for the following alignment: your elbows will be as close together as you can make them, that is, a shoulder's width apart. Your hands will be on your back as close to the shoulder blades as possible. This will prop your back straight into the air. As you progress in this pose you will experience the stretch originating from the base of your skull. Tuck your pelvis so that your pelvis will be aligned over your ribcage. Press your heels back so that your feet are over your buttocks. This will align you from the feet through to the shoulders the same as if you were standing, that is, the feet, pelvis, rib cage, and shoulders will be in a straight line. Push up out of your armpits to elongate the body, and press the balls of the feet toward the ceiling. You will find that your feet may rotate to the insides. This is because your large toes are lower than your small toes on a horizontal line. It then means that the insides of your thighs have shortened. This can be corrected by

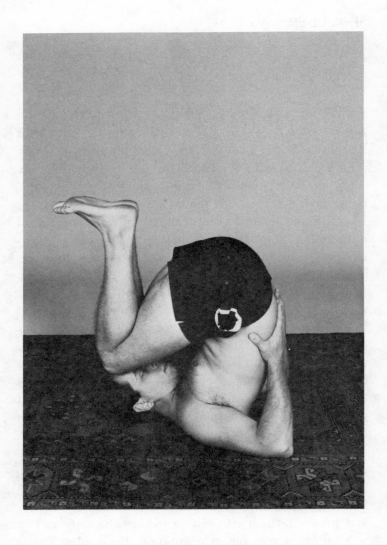

SHOULDERSTAND/ Step 1

pressing the balls behind your large toes up and towards the ceiling.

Some practitioners of yoga place a folded blanket or towel under their shoulders to preserve the cervical arch. If you are stiff, this is also a good thing to do. It will allow you to perform the posture to an extent that would typically be outside of your capacity.

If you are doing the entire series, go to the plow pose at this time by pulling your feet to the floor over the head. To come down, place your hands to the floor at the back, bending slightly at the hips, and slowly lower your body to the floor, one segment of the spine at a time.

If you are doing the shoulderstand only, then you must follow it with the fish pose.

Points to Notice: Be aware of your capacity while doing this pose. Take note of the pull in the shoulders and neck, and as you spend more time in the pose, notice if the tension at the neck and shoulders decreases. Later when you are able to maintain the shoulderstand for three minutes, you will find that the tension will be relieved by the end of the series.

Notice the draining of the blood from your feet and legs. As you progress with the posture, you will experience less and less discomfort associated with this draining. Your lower back may ache slightly. This too diminishes and disappears in time.

Make sure that the elbows stay as close in alignment with the shoulders as possible, as this will assist in keeping the body erect. Be sure that you continue to extend the body upward.

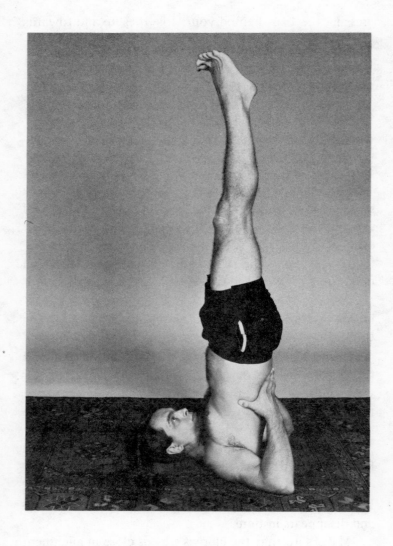

SHOULDERSTAND

Purpose: This posture has many benefits. The translation from its Sanskrit name *(sarvangasana)* means, "all limb pose," because it has impact throughout the body. I use it in therapy with specific intentions to effect stress management, strengthening the breathing systems, and affecting the circulation by turning the body upside down.

For stress management I use this posture with the plow to relieve tension in the shoulders and neck. For those with respiratory difficulty, this pose can prove very beneficial if done with caution. It slows the breath down and strengthens the diaphragm. When in the shoulderstand the weight of the liver, stomach, and intestines rests upon the diaphragm so that the diaphragm is required to work against this load during breathing. On the inhalation, when the diaphragm falttens, it has to raise the weight of the digestive system, much like a bench press. On the exhalation, the diaphragm must lower slower than usual to avoid collapsing under the weight of the digestive system. Those who lift free weights know that this negative weight lifting is where much of the strength is achieved.

I have found that this strengthening of the diaphragm in the shoulderstand has a major benefit for people with respiratory dysfunctions such as asthma. Inverted postures are also very beneficial for draining blood from the legs. For those who lead a sedentary life, the inverting postures serve as a very beneficial impact to the circulatory system.

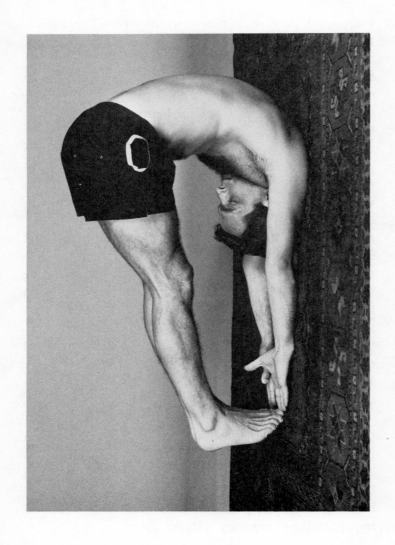

PLOW

PLOW

Technique: This posture can be done either from the shoulderstand or directly from lying on your back. If from lying on your back, exhale, lift the legs ninety degrees, and inhale. Then exhale, raise the legs over the head and lower your toes to the floor beyond your head. If done from the shoulderstand, exhale and lower your toes to the floor over your head.

To relieve pressure and make the pose easier, you can place your hands to the floor over your head at your feet. However, to gain additional benefit you can place your hands on the floor at the back side. Further benefit can be gained by joining the fingers together with the arms straight on the floor at the backside.

Proper performance of the posture will be achieved when the back is held straight from the shoulder all the way up to the end of the tailbone. To come out of the pose, lower the body to the floor one segment of the spine at a time, and go either to the bridge pose or the fish pose to complete the posture.

Points to Notice: Be aware of the accentuated pull at the neck, and continue to push the buttocks back so as to straighten the spine. This can be achieved once you acquire flexibility by pivoting the pelvis back where it connects at the lumbar. Press the torso up out of the armpits and press the arms and shoulders firmly to the floor. Be sure that the legs are kept straight. You can do this by pressing the backs of the knees toward the ceiling. Pull the chest further up, drawing the chin down toward the hollow of the neck. Remember to breathe.

Purpose: This posture accentuates the stress reduction benefits of relieving the neck and shoulders. It tends also to relieve the pressure on the skull.

I have found that once one becomes accustomed to this posture and the shoulderstand, there is a relaxation around the issues of claustrophobia and its accompanying psychological complement. I say this because many people experience a claustrophobic effect upon initially practicing these two postures.

The plow, when properly performed, dissipates rigidity in the lower back, buttocks, and hamstrings, and also is very beneficial for lower back pain.

BRIDGE

Technique: This posture can be done either from the floor or from the shoulderstand. From the floor, draw your heels in to the buttocks, hold onto the ankles with your hands, exhale and arch your pelvis up, keeping the syoulders and head on the floor.

A variation on this pose is achieved by arching the pelvis and back, placing your hands on the waist or hips rather than on the ankles.

From the shoulderstand, move the hands up to the waist or hips, and while exhaling, lower the feet to the floor one at a time, pivoting over your hands. Once the pose is achieved, tuck the pelvis firmly.

When you have held the pose to your capacity, lower the body to the floor. If your lower back feels uncomfortable, bend your knees and bring the bottoms of your feet to the floor. If you need more relief, hug your knees to your chest in order to stretch out the lower back.

Points to Notice: Be aware of your capacity while doing this pose. Tuck the pelvis to support the lower back and stretch the tops of the thighs open. Press the navel up toward the ceiling, roll the chest open at the shoulders, and push as to open the sternum. Breathe deeply so as to expand the chest. Spreading your knees and feet apart makes performance of the posture easier, and as you progress, bring your feet and knees closer together for maximum benefit. Upon coming down from the shoulderstand, move slowly, being very sensitive of your back.

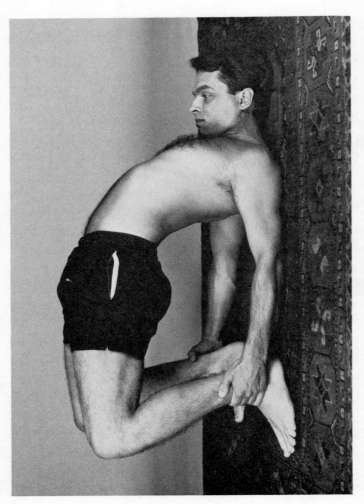

BRIDGE

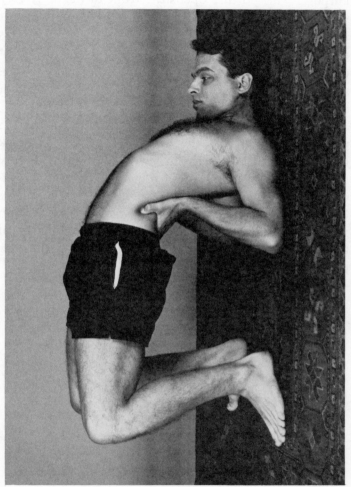

Purpose: This posture opens the front of the body very well by stretching it over the back side of the body. It also gradually gives a flexibility to the spine. This posture should be approached slowly, as should all of the postures, so that the opportunity for injury to oneself can be diminished significantly, if not altogether avoided.

One of the benefits of attitudes accompanying the yoga postures is that the awareness of the feedback that the physical organism gives is monitored very closely. This monitoring is done specifically to encounter what would previously be noted as unconscious behavior and signal systems. The signal systems also give subtle and gross data about the current limits of the body and can thus foretell stressing and straining parts of the body.

WHEEL

Caution: Be sure that your back is flexible and strong before attempting this pose. You need not be able to perform the posture perfectly, or even well, but you must not cause any injury to your back, arms, or neck. The wheel should be put in the shoulderstand series only after you have achieved a level of proficiency with the bridge and bow postures.

Technique: This posture can originate either from the floor or out of the bridge pose.

While on your back lying on the floor, bring your heels to your buttocks, exhale, and arch your pelvis and back from the floor. At this point all instructions will be the same whether going from the floor or out of the bridge. Bring the arms over the head, putting the palms of the hands to the floor by the ears, fingertips rotated back toward the heels. Be sure the pelvis is tucked. Inhale. Then exhale, pushing with the arms. Raise the head and shoulders off the floor. Tuck the pelvis, pushing the thighs and navel toward the ceiling. Breathe deeply. Stretch up out of the armpits and roll your chest open, pushing the arms and legs to straighter and straighter positions.

To lower as a part of the shoulderstand series, exhale, return to the bridge with the hands under the waist. To lower as a posture unto itself, lower the head, neck, and shoulders to the floor. Then place the buttocks to the floor and straighten the legs. If you need any relief for the lower back, bring the heels to the buttocks and bend the legs at the knees. If you need more relief, hug the knees to the chest.

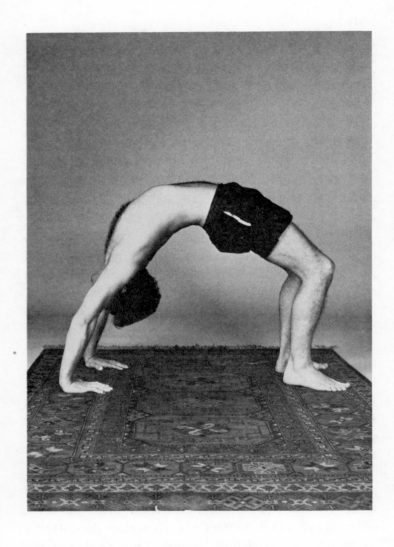

WHEEL

Points to Notice: Be aware of the lower back, ensuring that it is kept firm. Press the chest open. You may find that slowly putting your weight on your hands or shifting it to the feet will change the emphasis of the posture. Be sure to keep pressing the top of the thighs and the navel toward the ceiling and rotating the chest open.

Purpose: This posture even more dramatically works on opening the front of the body. People who perform it very easily and yet are not able to bend the other way, are probably not able to establish their limits, nor have a clear sense of their boundaries, but rather allow others to manipulate them. Those who are flexible in both directions I would initially consider to be balanced. If a person has a weak front but is weak in the arms and shoulders, they may not be able to get to the point for you to observe them.

Be careful about being too ready to judge based on this bias because there will be a great number of people who would not have the frontal flexibility to open themselves up in this posture. For these I would investigate a willingness to be vulnerable. Again remember that in the maturation of the human ego it is the assemblage and eventual transcendence of defense mechanisms that create the stages of human development. What you have provided is the context whereby individuals can encounter the self-established boundaries that have served them well up to that point. You have introduced a "choice point" whereby they can reconsider whether or not this current limit continues to serve them in their growth.

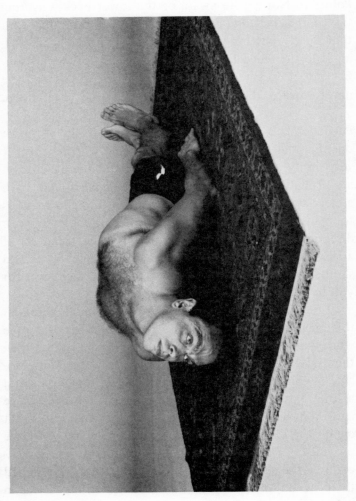

FISH

FISH

Technique: This posture can be done of itself or be used as the end in the shoulderstand series. In both cases your body will be lying flat on the floor in the corpse pose to begin.

While lying on your back, keep your legs straight and arch your chest up, keeping your buttocks to the floor. In arching, place the top of the head to the floor. The hands are to remain on the floor at your sides, or rest on the tops of your thighs. The front of the throat is to be stretched as far as possible.

Points to Notice: Be aware of the breath and stretch the rib cage open with each breath. Open your chest, and press with your back as if the spine were to push the sternum up out of the chest.

Purpose: This pose gives the neck the opposite bend from the shoulderstand and plow, and opens the throat and chest where repression may be harbored.

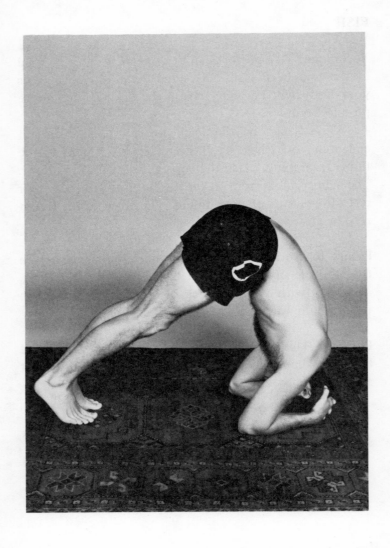

HEADSTAND / Step 1

HEADSTAND

Caution: Here is a test to ensure that your neck muscles are strong enough for this posture: Lie on your back, arms by your side. While keeping your shoulders to the floor, raise your head as high as you can and have a second person gently, yet firmly, press against your head in the direction of the floor, with the heel of his hand at your forehead. You should resist as much as you can. If your head moves toward the floor with little resistance, then your neck and shoulder muscles are not strong enough for this posture, and the dolphin pose should be practiced to strengthen the neck.

You may want to start practicing the headstand six to twelve inches away from a wall for security. In my yoga classes, however, I encourage people to learn without a wall. In a therapeutic context where the intent is not necessarily directed toward achieving the full outcomes of hatha yoga, I recommend the use of the wall for beginners.

Technique: Kneeling, sit to your heels, join your fingers and place your hands to the floor eighteen inches in front of your knees. Spread your elbows the width of your shoulders apart, and place the top of your head on the floor with the back of your head in the hollow created by your hands. Your hands will be in a position whereby the small fingers will be on the floor and the fingers will be stacked with thumbs on top.

Come up onto the balls of your feet and raise your buttocks in the air. This will create a triangle from your head to your hips to your feet. Walk your legs in toward the chest until your weight moves onto your forearms

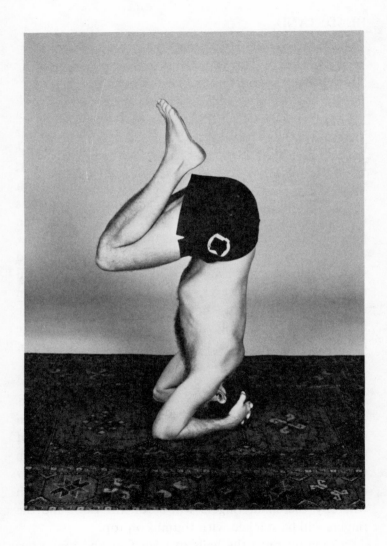

HEADSTAND / Step 2

and head.

Shifting your weight to your head and arms, balance, and bring your knees into your chest, raising your feet off the floor and tucking them in toward the buttocks. Pause here and check your balance.

Slowly raise your legs toward the ceiling until your legs are straightened overhead. The alignment will be the same as when you are standing. The head, shoulders, pelvis, and ankles will all be smoothly aligned. The weight is to be distributed on the elbows, forearms, wrists, hands, and head. You can tell that you have achieved a level of competency when there is a comfortable sense of weightlessness in the posture. If you are using the wall, use it only to steady yourself with your heel when necessary. Other than that, stay free of the wall, and balance on your forearms and head.

Points to Notice: Be aware of your internal dialogue associated with going into and maintaining this posture. If you are not initially successful in the pose, reasons why you should not be or will not be will surface in the form of internal dialogue, pictures of failure, or uncomfortable sensations in the body. If this is the case, rehearse successful performance in these three channels in your imagination.

Be sure that you continue to distribute your weight into the forearms, head, and elbows. If you tend to go over backwards or fall back to the front, this means that you are putting too much weight on the head or the elbows respectively, and need to adjust your pelvis more accurately over your shoulders.

Be mindful of the breath and keep the abdomen and pelvis firm so that the legs, which are also kept firm, can

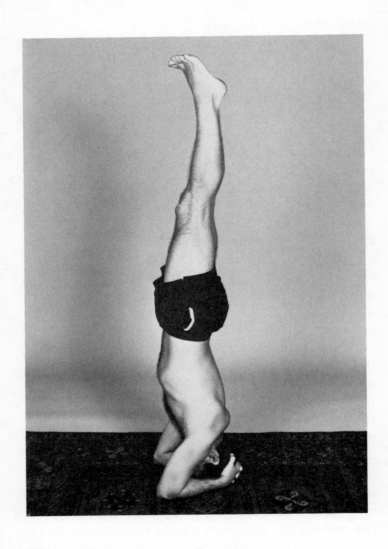

HEADSTAND

be controlled while in the air. If you relax your abdomen and lower back when first learning this posture, you may find it difficult to perform. As you become more adept, you can begin to release unnecessary tensions in your system. Push up out of the armpits and the base of your skull. Tuck your pelvis, aligning it over the chest, and push your heels back over your buttocks.

Purpose: This posture reveals a lot to me. My experience in therapy and years of yoga classes have supported the following bias. If a person takes over and above the typical learning period to master this pose, I begin to explore his issues around experiencing life outside of the confines of his current reality. I have found such people to have a very narrow range that they define as secure and comfortable. Seeing life and the things of life from a different perspective is something they are not basically willing to do. We all have degrees of this, but some people are extreme in their avoidance of what is "other than usual" from their perspective. By overtly shifting their relationship with the external reality, they experience an inordinate amount of anxiety.

Most people will experience some anxiety associated with inverting the body and balancing on their head. This is due to the fear associated with moving outside of the known. But it is eventually encountered and overcome. Thus I use this piece of data as a signal that I need to explore risk-taking, security, and self-assertiveness with the individual. This posture totally changes a person's relationships to his world by 180 degrees.

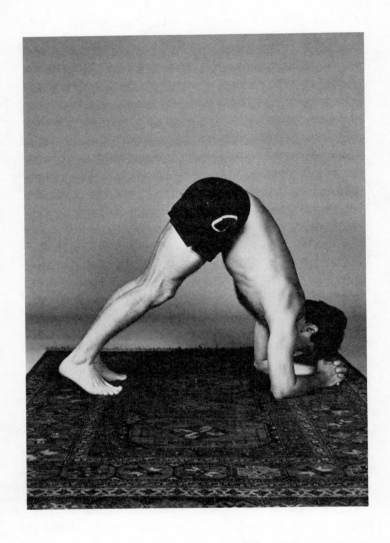

DOLPHIN

DOLPHIN

Technique: Kneeling, sit to your heels, lock your fingers together, and place them to the floor eighteen inches in front of your knees. Rest your weight on your forearms. Bringing the balls of your feet to the floor, raise your hips in the air, straightening your legs. This will create a triangle with your elbows, hips, and feet. Your head is to be held off the floor and raised so that you are facing the floor the entire length of the exercise.

Points to Notice: Be aware of the strength of your shoulders and the strength of the back of the neck in this posture.

Purpose: This posture strengthens the muscles of the neck in preparation for the headstand. It will also address issues of self-support associated with the shoulders and the frontal muscles of the neck.

10
Relaxation

It is difficult, if not impossible, to instruct someone in how to relax. When someone *tries* to relax, the organism ends up moving into a state contradictory to the request. Relaxation is, by definition, absence of effort. Therefore we are not, strictly speaking, instructing in how to relax because doing requires effort.

Relaxation is the natural state of the body when it is left to its own devices. This is a creative position producing desired outcomes. When the organism is stimulated, it moves into a state of effort to produce an outcome currently not being generated in homeostasis.

Thus parts of the body are brought into a state of tension or activity. This is also a creative position producing desired outcomes. Hence tension and relaxation can both be highly desirable states. It is a matter of choice.

In a therapeutic setting we encourage clients to choose by giving them additional choices to make. If one is in a state of relaxation and cannot choose something else, we would call that paralysis. If one were in a state of tension and could not choose something else, we would call that a state of anxiety. The dysfunction comes from choicelessness.

The power of relaxation exercises lies in the ability to leave the body alone. Most people do not know how to "let alone," so we guide them into a state of tension and then request that they release. Relaxation naturally follows.

In a therapeutic setting I find it particularly essential to address issues of accumulated stress. The nervous system is by nature a design for coping with stress. Basically, when an emergency presents itself the autonomic nervous system shifts from maintenance of health to the protection of the organism. This design is developed to provide, under emergency conditions, the shifting of resources (such as blood flow, oxygen intake, glucose breakdown, and brain stimulation) from housekeeping to military alert.*

Due to the interaction with group members and therapists, a client's persona in therapy is put under scrutiny. While this is done for psychological growth

* For more information on this topic see *Freedom from Stress* by Phil Nuernberger, Ph.D. (Honesdale, PA: Himalayan Press, 1982).

and development, the anxiety associated with such scrutiny can send hormonal secretion into the blood stream of the client, causing the nervous system to switch to a state of alert. I will refer to this point as arousal peaking. It is a natural response of the nervous system, and once the cause of the stimulus is resolved, the nervous system will naturally return to a state of ease. What we find in therapy, as well as in everyday life, is that these stimulators do not have immediate or clear-cut resolutions. In our modern day life, as well as in therapy, the nervous system must be given assistance in achieving a rebound of relaxation from the arousal peaking.

The relaxation exercises of yoga lend themselves very profoundly to this end. For the nervous system it matters not whether the problem is resolved. To regain physiological health associated with stress, what matters is that the nervous system be allowed to move back into the maintenance category for a period of time. Then it can, according to design, return to a state of arousal so that the additional resources available in that state can again be applied for creative problem solving. The difficulty of stress is that when one is in a state of unregulated arousal, one's creativity diminishes significantly, in part due to the incapability of the organism to function clearly over long periods in the emergency mode.

Another value that relaxation has for therapy is that it brings about the opportunity to contact the natural body. The body in a state of arousal is, of course, a natural body, but it is a body in reaction to emergency. What we hope to produce is a body moving at its own rhythm. By that I mean the synchronization of heart rate, breath, hormone secretion, gastro-intestinal function, muscle tone, and priority of blood flow distribution. The human body is of itself the space where transformation comes into existence. If one can leave the body alone, it is the natural climate for self-realization.

This knowledge is very valuable in furthering the understanding of unconscious behavior, and also the ability to be fully present in one's body. I find this access to unconscious behavior (for example, heart rate, respiration rate, hormonal secretion, and intestinal stimulation) an important element in self-transformation.

Behavior is both psychologically and physiologically based. The largest portion of behavior is unconscious, first in its origin and second in its execution. By deepening the awareness of, and sensitivity to, a structure of behavior, we have a greater portion of the person to work with in any therapeutic setting. By easing the nervous system, relaxation exercises are valuable for loosening or opening up the defense mechanisms. As a result of systematically and creatively opening the defense mechanisms, intervention can be instituted in a much shorter time frame, and with more conscious participation on the part of the client.

Another value for the relaxation exercises is as a transitional mechanism from whatever activities the clients were involved in before our session, to the work that I have scheduled. I have found this especially helpful when working with teenagers and children in assisting them to calm down for the type of work that is to follow.

How to Lead a Relaxation Exercise

How one delivers the relaxation exercise can have a significant impact upon the effect the exercise has on the recipient. First, it is important to acknowledge yourself as a coach, realizing that the features of the relaxation must show up in the client. You will be, on the one hand, pointing out directions to be explored, and on the other hand, reminding the relaxing person to stay on task. The following are some guidelines in leading a relaxation.

Voice Quality

Voice quality is extremely important in leading group relaxations. Conduct the following experiment to experience this fact for yourself. Say, "Be aware of the breath flowing through your nostrils." Say this four times, and each time listen to the quality of your voice, noticing if there is any mood shift in your intent. The first time, say the sentence while focusing your attention in your abdomen. Second, say the sentence while focusing in the center of your chest. Third, say it when focusing in your throat. Last, say the sentence while focusing in your head. I have found that I have a greater sense of ease in delivery and a more positive response from clients when I focus in the center of my chest cavity.

Speed

There are two factors in speed: the pace of delivery and the space between each delivery. In the pace of delivery the rate of speaking should be slightly slower than that used in conversational speech, yet at the same time it should not be overly affective. Upon delivery it should seem that you are speaking conversationally, but by comparison, in the context of relaxation, the pace will be a lot slower. Also . . . in the pace of delivery . . . you might consider . . . breaking up your sentences . . . into . . . smaller segments . . . so that subconscious understanding . . . will be able . . . to totally translate . . . your requests. As you can see by this example, you add a richness to what you are saying by creating subphrases with the pauses that you insert in the sentence. Be mindful not to overdo this and become monotonous. This is another way to say "be creative."

In creating spaces after each delivery, you should likewise give the recipient time to be aware of the experience to which you are pointing. This is very important. If you give too much time, the mind will become bored and drift into fantasy. Perfect timing will develop with performance.

Volume

It is important to speak loud enough so as to be heard by everyone in the group. As you become more skillful, you can actually give a relaxation exercise to a mass of people speaking at the top of your voice. So it is not necessary to whisper. A general rule that I follow in establishing rapport in relaxation is to begin speaking loudly, but below lecturing volume. As I sense the relaxation taking place, I follow suit by progressively softening my voice. I may even end up in a whisper so as not to disturb the sensitive state that has been brought about.

Reminders

You are, in effect, the clients' conscience when

leading a relaxation exercise. You assist them in remaining on task by occasionally inserting statements of reminders, such as:

"If you find that you are translating your experiences into words, let go of them and return your awareness to . . . " (whatever part of the body or activity you are dealing with at the time).

"As we travel you will come into contact with memories. Rather than commenting to yourself upon these memories, pass through them, continuing to attend to . . . " or

"If you have an idea as to how this part is supposed to be, let go of that idea and be aware of how it is."

Crutches

If you give relaxation exercises often it is important to be aware of personal idiosyncracies that may distract others. Have someone critique you, since most probably you will not be able to notice these behaviors yourself. They usually occur at points when you are thinking what to say next, though they are not limited to these times. Some common crutches in speaking are listed here:

1. Periodic clearing of the throat.
2. Saying "um" or "you know" between phrases.
3. Adding OK between sentences.
4. Raising your voice at the end of every sentence.
5. Drumming your fingers on the podium.
6. Lingering on the last syllable of the sentence.
7. Pulling at an earlobe or touching some part of the face.

These are only examples which do not exhaust the list of possible crutches. If you have a group of people who hear you often they will begin to notice your crutch and be distracted either by aggravation or by humor.

Posture

As you deliver a relaxation exercise, the way in which you sit or stand will impact your voice quality. Your personal experience of relaxation will always be conveyed in your voice as well as your posture. People most probably will not be sensitive to this consciously, but will most definitely know it at other-than-conscious levels, and will react. If someone is peeking, seeing you wringing your hands will cause you to lose a little credibility.

How to End a Relaxation Exercise

The ending of a relaxation exercise needs to be sensitively and skillfully handled. Remember that since you are coaching your intention is to create your work so that the client no longer needs you for the particular skill you are delivering. I would like to point out here the importance of repetition. By doing the same thing over and over again without any changes the other-than-conscious part of the mind will master the task.

Upon giving a relaxation exercise, you have brought the client to a very sensitive state in regard to his nervous system. It is important to prepare the nervous system for reentry to the typical impact level of sensory experience. There are a number of ways to do this, one of which is as follows:

As you come out, bring your hands before your eyes. Open your eyes into your hands so that your hands are the first things that you see when you open your eyes. Slowly lower

your hands to your sides and with your
eyes open know that you understand everything before you, but be free from changing
your experience into words. Be with the
experience as it is. Continue to attend to your
breath. At some point when you feel inclined,
release, and come to an upright position.

I emphasize "open your eyes" because it is an em-
bedded command. You have already made the request
to come out of the relaxation. This emphasis on opening
the eyes is an additional request to those who are
choosing to stay in the relaxation longer. This will roust
them out. I say the word "release" at the end just in
case anyone has gone into a hypnotic trance. This, then,
is a command for them to release connection to any
suggestion that might have triggered a deep trance state.

The following relaxation exercises are based upon
classical yogic methods of sense withdrawal. I suggest
that you do not embellish them. They can be used as a
prelude, if you wish, to one of your creative adventures,
but they should not be changed. There is nothing sacred
about the following exercises, but as they stand, they
work.

Postures for Relaxation

There are two postures that are appropriate for
relaxation. They are the corpse pose and the friendship pose. Guide your clients into one of these postures
at the beginning of each relaxation exercise.

THE CORPSE POSE

Technique: Sitting down on the floor, lie backwards, lengthening your spine by stretching the vertebra, placing them to the floor one at a time. Finally place the back of your head to the floor after lengthening the neck. Spread your arms about ten inches from the torso or until you can rest the back of the hands on the floor, palms up, without any effort in the upper arms or shoulders. Spread your legs about two feet apart. Allow your feet to fall to the outsides and release any effort in the body. Close your eyes and breathe abdominally.

Points to Notice: Be aware of the level of comfort in this pose. Notice especially any discomfort in the lower back. Feel free to bend your legs at the knees and rest the bottoms of the feet on the floor. This will relieve pressure and strain on the lower back. You can maintain this position for as long as is necessary to relieve the discomfort in the back.

Purpose: There are a number of agendas associated with this posture. To assume this pose requires a high degree of trust because the front of the body is totally exposed. If a client has difficulty with this level of vulnerability, he will not be able to close his eyes. In a sense he will have to keep an eye on everything. It is important to appreciate the level of trust that is assumed when you request someone to assume this pose.

You can also observe ego strength through body tone by observing how close the feet rotate out to the floor. Unless an individual has gone through much training, such as dance, to achieve a "turn out," his thighs will not rotate so that the outsides of the feet can touch the floor. My bias is to explore for depth of ego strength here. Has he defined himself to himself? Typically babies will lack definition in the groin and thigh because they have not encountered life in a way that would have a reflexive response in this region. Thus their feet will quite easily fall over to the side. A point of interest is when I see someone who looks infantile, adolescent, or even pre-adolescent when in his thirties or forties, I ask myself why he inhabits his body in this fashion and at what point did his maturation process halt?

THE FRIENDSHIP POSE

Technique: Sitting in a chair with your head, neck, and trunk erect, rest your hands on your lap and place your feet squarely on the floor about a foot apart. Let your breath be abdominal.

Points to Notice: Be aware that your spine is kept erect and that your head remains balanced over your rib cage so that tension does not develop in the neck and shoulder area.

Purpose: This pose is typically used for relaxation when the environment is not conducive for lying down in the corpse pose. It would be applicable in an office setting, in an environment where furniture would interfere with the posture, or for those who have a disability and are unable to lie on their back.

RELAXATION EXERCISE 1
Tension / Relaxation

In this exercise you will be asked to isolate body parts and then scan the rest of the body. This is a mental survey of the other body parts to ensure that they are not tensing sympathetically. There is a high tendency for some limbs, or even the face, to tense in sympathy with another limb, just like a mother opening her mouth while spoon-feeding her child.

The isolation will heighten the faculty of discrimination by drawing sharper distinctions. In isolation be sure that the tensed limb is not raised off the floor, because in order to raise the limb, you must also tense the adjoining large muscle group, thus interfering with the discriminative element we are striving for. This distinction may require a redefinition of tension to complement the goal of self-exploration and transformation. Tension does not have to be rock-hard solidity of muscles. It can exist even at the level of an idea or an intention. The point is that the limb should be tense, but it does not have to be rigid. In rigidity there always is spillover into other muscle groups.

The instruction to release is a request to "let go" of muscular tension and experience the response that that limb is producing in its released state, be it visual, kinesthetic, and/or auditory. If you find sympathetic release taking place in another limb, you were holding tension unconsciously and are being signalled. This is a further sensitizing toward dialogue between the conscious and other-than-conscious parts of the mind.

Technique: While lying in the corpse pose:

Turn your right palm to the floor.

Tense your right arm.

Scan and isolate.

Release.

Turn your right palm up.

Turn your left palm to the floor.

Tense your left arm.

Scan and isolate.

Release.

Turn your left palm up.

Tense the right leg (do not tense the buttock).

Scan and isolate.

Release.

Tense the left leg (do not tense the buttock).

Scan and isolate.

Release.

Turn your right palm to the floor.

Tense your right arm and right leg.

Scan and isolate.

Release.

Turn your right palm up.

Turn your left palm to the floor.

Tense your left arm and left leg.

Scan and isolate.

Release.

Turn your left palm up.

Turn your right and left palms to the floor.

Tense your right and left arms.

Scan and isolate.

Release.

Turn your palms up.

Tense your right and left legs, including the buttocks.

Scan and isolate.

Release.

During one of your inhalations, progressively tense the body from the toe tips to the crown of the head. Coincide maximum inhalation with maximum tension. Hold the tension for a short period of time. You may, if you wish, hold the breath for five to ten seconds before you release, if you do not have any physical disorder that breath retention would aggravate (such as high blood pressure, epilepsy, heart disorders, asthma, etc.). Exhale and release the tension with the outflow of breath. Lie in this state, being aware of the spectrum of the unconscious movement in the nervous system, be it auditory, kinesthetic, or visual. Come out slowly.

RELAXATION EXERCISE 2
Be Aware

This exercise gives an experience of how to leave the body alone, and at the same time be fully cognizant of the nature of our individual perception.

When moving through this exercise you will be requested to be aware of specific segments of the body. Be very clear that you are to do nothing to that part of the body except be fully involved in the experience. If you at all have a preconception of how that particular part is supposed to be, or experience a desire to shift that part of the body, do not fulfill that desire. Leave the body alone. Know each part of the body as the experience that comes forward. My intention in using this exercise is to let each part of the body teach itself to you.

Remember to attend to voice quality, pace, and the space between each request. Add any of the following questions at points during the exercise as reminders to observe the body:

"Are you seeing the experience?"

"Are you feeling the experience?"

"Are you hearing the experience?"

"If you feel, do you experience this body part (for example, the arm) as lying on a plane higher or lower than the other?"

This questioning acquaints the client with his method of gathering information about the current experience.

Be sure to instruct the clients in how to lie in the corpse pose each time you use it. In the following exercise it is vital to allow sufficient time to elapse between directions for the client to neurologically identify his responses.

Technique: While lying in the corpse pose,

Be aware of your head.

Now your shoulders.

Now your arms.

Now your hands.

Now be aware of your pelvis.

Now your legs.

Now your feet.

Be aware of the breath moving the abdomen.

Experience the rise and the fall of the abdomen.

If you find the breath long, be aware of its length.

If you find the breath short, be aware of its shortness.

Be aware now of its depth or its shallowness, its raggedness or its smoothness.

Let the breath alone.

Let the breath breathe your body.
Be aware of the breath passing through your nostrils.
Be aware of the warmth of the exhalation.
Be aware of the coolness of the inhalation.
Rather than trying to make more breath pass through
  your nostrils,
Be aware of the breath that is already there.
Be aware of the crown of your head.
As you exhale, travel to the toetips.
As you inhale, travel to the crown of the head.
Exhale and inhale between these two points.
  (Let this be done for a period of time.)
Return the awareness to the breath at the nostrils,
  exhaling and inhaling.

At this point you could end the relaxation, or continue
into Relaxation Exercise 3.

RELAXATION EXERCISE 3
Body and Breath Awareness

In addition to the experience of deep relaxation that
this exercise provides, it creates an opportunity for
being in the present, and for experiencing responses to
different parts of the body. Two points are important
here. First, remember to give the occasional reminder
for people may drift into fantasy. You may request that
clients note over the weeks if similar types of fantasies
are generated at the same parts of the body each time
they perform the exercise. Second, some people may
move into an unconscious state during the exercise. We
call that sleep. In yoga, sleep is referred to as the absence

of cognition. This points out that there is not an absence of a phenomenon, but for a rational mind there is an absence of knowing the phenomenon. In the relaxation exercise you are guiding the individual through the dream state. Sometimes in this travel one can come close enough to unconscious realms to occasionally drift into the state of sleep. You may even hear people snore. What is interesting to note, however, is that upon the request to the group to come out of relaxation, those who demonstrated deep sleep behavior come out on cue. This is an indication that they were processing what was taking place in the session, but were at the same time functioning in a realm outside of their awareness.

During the course of this exercise, give the client time to exhale and inhale between the two points at least once. You may want to use some of the following statements:

"Exhale and inhale betwen these two points at the rate of the breath until we move to the next part of the exercise."

"However long it takes you to exhale, use that time to travel to . . . ."

"However long it takes you to inhale, use that time to return to the crown of the head."

"If by chance you find that you are talking to yourself about the memories you most assuredly will come into contact with, let go of that and return the awareness to the breath."

These will encourage them not to shorten the breath to correspond to the distance from one body part to the crown of the head, as well as to keep their attention on the task at hand.

Technique: Lying in the corpse pose,
Bring the awareness to the crown of the head.
As you exhale, travel to the toe tips.
As you inhale, travel to the crown of the head.
As you exhale, travel to the feet.
As you inhale, travel to the crown of the head.
As you exhale, travel to the calf muscles.
As you inhale, travel to the crown of the head.
As you exhale, travel to the thighs.
As you inhale, travel to the crown of the head.
As you exhale, travel to the pelvis.
As you inhale, travel to the crown of the head.
As you exhale, travel to the base of the spine.
As you inhale, travel to the crown of the head.
As you exhale, travel to the navel.
As you inhale, travel to the crown of the head.
As you exhale, travel to the center of the chest.
As you inhale, travel to the crown of the head.
As you exhale, travel to the hollow of the neck.
As you inhale, travel to the crown of the head.
Bring the awareness to the forehead at the center
    between the eyebrows.
During the exhalation, travel to the point where the
    nostrils meet the upper lip.
During the inhalation, travel to the center between the
    eyebrows. Exhale and inhale, moving back and
    forth between these two points at the rate of the
    breath. (Let clients do this for a period of time,
    reminding them occasionally to be aware of the
    breath either auditorially, kinesthetically, or visually.
    "Do you hear the breath, feel the breath, or see the
    breath?"
Bring the awareness to the crown of the head.

During exhalation, extend the awareness to the hollow of the neck.

During inhalation, travel to the crown of the head.

During exhalation, extend the awareness to the center of the chest.

During inhalation, travel to the crown of the head.

During exhalation, extend the awareness to the navel.

During inhalation, travel to the crown of the head.

During exhalation, extend the awareness to the base of the spine.

During inhalation, travel to the crown of the head.

During exhalation, extend the awareness to the pelvis.

During inhaaltion, travel to the crown of the head.

During exhalation, extend the awareness to the thighs.

During inhalation, travel to the crown of the head.

During exhalation, extend the awareness to the calf muscles.

During inhalation, travel to the crown of the head.

During exhalation, extend the awareness to the feet.

During inhalation, travel to the crown of the head.

During exhalation, extend the awareness to the toetips.

During inhalation, travel to the crown of the head.

Exhaling and inhaling, breathe with your entire body.

Bring the awareness to the forehead at the center between the eyebrows.

Exhale, and travel to the point where the nostrils meet the upper lip.

Inhale, and travel to the center between the eyebrows.

Exhale back and forth between these two points.

Come out slowly.

11
Breathing

The yogic sages looked into the seed of human existence and found the fulcrum upon which life is balanced. They discovered, through experiments on themselves and others, that the breath is the crucial link between body and mind. In their investigation they found, very simply speaking, that humans could live weeks without food, days without water, but only minutes without breath.

The breath links all breathing creatures to the outside environment and to each other because all are involved in the cycle of exhalation and inhalation.

All breathe the same air.

The sages noticed that any motion in the mind influenced the breath, and was subtly connected to the body through the breath. They found that the breath reflects the mind, and that one can affect the mind by the breath. This discovery opened for them an opportunity to impact mental and emotional environments for the self-transformative work that has been passed down from teacher to student for thousands of years. According to master yogi, Swami Rama,

> When the student comes in touch with the finer forces called prana (the energy of the breath) he can learn to control his mind, for it is tightly fastened to the prana like a kite to a string. When the string is held skillfully, the kite, which wants to fly here and there, is controlled and flies in the direction desired. . . . He who has controlled his breath has also controlled his mind. He who has controlled his mind has also controlled his breath.*

Let us point out what is meant by the word "control" in this context. Control means "to direct" exactly the way the banks of a river direct the flow of water. If the water were to overflow the banks it would become a flood and be destructive to life. When the water is controlled by the river banks it becomes a life-giving source to the environment. So we are speaking here of control as a creative act, not as an act of suppression.

Yogis do not suppress their emotions, but they do control them. In addition to other techniques (i.e., meditation, body work, willingness to live with the

* Swami Rama, et al. *Science of Breath*. (Honesdale, PA: Himalayan Press, 1979) 91-92.

unknown, skillful action, using the past as a resource rather than as a dictum or a hiding place, and so forth), yogis use breathing practices to increase the capacity of the nervous system to tolerate emotional charge. They thus allow the personality to function with their current level of wisdom while experiencing the intensity of the emotion. They can then explore, with intelligence and clarity of mind, the opportunity to feel fully, and at the same time be in partnership with the rational mind, as well as the access that the rational mind has to the newest levels of insight.

Our breath directly and indirectly effects and is effected by our defense mechanisms. Human beings have an instinctual response to hold the breath and tighten all flexor muscles at the initial emergency of danger. Moshe Felderkris says of an infant,

> . . . if suddenly lowered, or if support is sharply withdrawn, a violent contraction of all flexors with halt of breath is observed, followed by crying, accelerated pulse and general vasomotor disturbance.

He states that this response in an infant is very similar to that of an adult in fear.

> The attitude of fear, the sinking of the head, the crouching, the bending of the knees, etc. . . are but details of the general contraction of all flexor muscles compatible with the act of standing.*

In like manner, Dr. Alexander Lowen in his book, *The Betrayal of the Body* points out how a schizoid

* Moshe Feldenkrais, *Body and Mature Behavior, A Study of Anxiety, Sex, Gravitation and Learning (New York: International Universities Press, Inc., 1975)* 84.

locks tension into his diaphragm and abdominal muscles as a strategy to insulate against experiencing sensations in the abdominal and pelvic regions associated with sex, fear, and bodily functions, among others.

We see here modern confirmation of what the yogis who studied the breath discovered: that breathing, and the anatomy associated with the breath, is very closely related to thoughts and feelings in the mind. Breathing is a most vital diagnostic tool for insight into developmental transformation. Knowledge of the language of the breath—its rhythm, speed, sound, depth, or any inhibition of its natural flow—is essential for therapeutic intervention. Stopping this natural flow, regardless of the extent, creates dysfunction both physically and emotionally. In daily life we come into contact with people who are fearful, joyful, angry, sad, loving, or fearless. All of these emotions are directly related to the way one breathes. The yogic breathing techniques and practices were devised to reinstate the natural flow of the breath, which is a context wherein emotional maturity can come into existence.

In my work in individual counseling, as well as in family or group sessions, I find that when a client has difficulty in gaining access to an emotion it is helpful to have him begin to breathe more deeply, focusing his emphasis on abdominal breathing right there in my office. This allows the motion of the experience to pass through his body more easily, providing an opportunity for him to consciously communicate with and about the experience in a therapeutic setting.

Breathing is primarily an other-than-conscious function. As we have seen, human behavior has an unconscious mechanism for defending itself physically and emotionally. Through interrupting, interferring with, or diminishing the breath, we can appear to hold our emotions at bay by keeping them outside of our awareness. If tools are not developed to manage these emotions they will eventually stack up into an unmanageable pile of fear and pain.

It is important to realize that this strategy of repression is passed on to the species in our genes. We employ it consciously. The yogic sages say breath is life, so if one judges it necessary to diminish the experience of life (through fear of the experience), one can diminish breath and ignore life's intensity. Thus it is essential in the developmental work of therapy to reintegrate fully breathing beings. One must choose to breathe again and thus experience life.

By allowing the breath to flow naturally, one experiences the depth of feeling associated with mature living. At the same time one uses the breath to feel more deeply, one also uses the breath to give guidance and direction to the emotions. One is therefore no longer a fish tossed about on the sea of emotion.

There was a client in a drug treatment center who had to attend an upcoming judicial hearing which would determine whether or not he would serve a jail sentence, or be allowed to go on parole and complete his drug treatment therapy. Bob was thirty-seven years old at the time, and had a history of rebellion against institutional authority. He had had numerous run-ins with police and the judicial system. He would be belligerent and abusive in court, which made his case so much worse. He was unaware of the complex wave of neurological responses that he linguistically interpreted as fear followed by defiance when he was in the presence of a judge.

At this time I began working with Bob, teaching him even breathing and breath awareness techniques. Soon he was able to experience and discriminate for the first time the feelings which arose in him. On the day he went to the court to determine his final eligibility, he remained conscious of his bodily responses, acknowledged his feelings, and yet was clear enough to serve his needs in a more mature fashion by conversing with the presiding judge as adult to adult. This change in behavior impressed the judge enough to warrant treatment and parole rather than jail. Bob told me later that the only thing he did different this time was breathe. He was then able to access resources already available within himself, together with those he had learned in therapy, to do what was necessary.

Breath is so vital and so powerful a tool that I would like to have you experience its power. Therefore I make a challenge to you: make this information about breathing very real for yourself by conducting an experiment. Practice the complete breath (see p. 307) for five minutes three times a day for three months (although one month will give you significant outcome), and see what happens for you.

Implementing the breath as a key to development is vital to assure that the human organism is functioning effectively, according to design, and is thus available to the full experience of life as it is presented. An integrated, conscious being is the context where curiosity, fearlessness, learning, growth, and assimilation take place. Transformation then naturally shows up in this context. Knowledge is the fruit of this integration.

How to Breathe

It is very important, even essential, to study the breath, although breathing is something we do naturally every moment of our life. We have so interfered with the natural design of breathing through prolonged stress and anxiety, bad habits, and ignorance that we must ask the question, What is normal breathing? Let us take a closer look at the process of breathing in order to understand the impact of the practices which follow.

Anatomy and Physiology

To begin we will assume that the body is in the natural or relaxed position of exhalation with the glottis open. The lungs and stomach share the same opening—the throat. The glottis is designed to close off the trachea when swalloring to prevent those contents destined for the stomach from getting into the lungs. Coughing is the body's attempt to expel foreign substances from the lungs; choking occurs when the glottis does not shut off the bypass to the lungs correctly, allowing particles to block or stimulate constriction of the breath passage.

The contents of the chest are wrapped in a membrane forming an airtight seal around the lungs and heart. The walls of the chest are constructed of the flexible bones of the rib cage. The partition that separates the chest from the abdominal cavities is called the diaphragm. It serves as both the floor of the chest cavity and the roof of the abdominal cavity. The abdominal cavity and its contents are also wrapped, like the chest cavity, in a membrane that forms an airtight seal around its contents. In this way, as will be explained later, a movement in one cavity can effect the other. The digestive system, which passes through these two cavities, does not interrupt their integrity or break their seal. We actually have an outer skin and an inner skin, like a tube running the length of the torso. Food goes into the mouth and passes through the body and out the rectum. The body then takes the nutrition it needs through the walls of the gastro-intestinal tract.

All cells of the body need oxygen in order to function. Breathing supplies oxygen to the circulatory system by way of respiration. Oxygen is required to mix with the fuel to provide combustion (at a slow rate in the body) needed to release energy in the cells. Dr. Alan Hymes, a cardiovascular and thoracic surgeon says,

> The actual process of respiration occurs within the cell where nutrient fuel is burned with oxygen to release energy. The nose, trachea (windpipe), lungs, circulatory system, and their attendant muscles all act to transport or modify O_2 from the surrounding air to make it really available to individual cells within the body. Each of these organs plays a crucial role in determining oxygen supply, and therefore energy availability, to cells at various levels within the body. A change in functioning in any one of these systems could therefore potentially alter the course of energy production within the body.*

In light of this it is important to be aware of the connection between lungs and heart. The body requires, depending upon energy needs, specific amounts of oxygenated blood. If correct breathing (which would deliver the demanded oxygen) is not implemented, the heart must then pump more blood through the portion

* Swami Rama, et al., op cit., 28.

of the lungs being ventilated in order to meet that need. This requires the heart to work many times harder than it would have to under full ventilation. Thus the work of the heart increases or decreases by the efficiency of breathing. Stress-related breathing, if employed over a long period of time, can overwork the heart muscle, especially if a poor diet clogs the arteries preventing the heart itself from receiving proper nutrition and oxygen content.

At this point it is important to look at one of the vital links in the breathing cycle: the nostrils. Most of us are familiar with the nasal functions of cleaning, moistening, cooling, and heating of inhaled air and the retrieving of body heat from exhaled air. Based on these functions alone, the value of the nostrils is quite evident. But there are many other functions of the nostrils which we shall point out.

The nostrils should be used for all breathing except in special cases. It is sometimes thought that when oxygen needs have increased, the mouth should be used to meet these needs. However, Dr. Justin O'Brien, in his book *Running and Breathing* says that even for the strenuous activity of running, nostril breathing can and should be employed.*

One of the chief functions of the nostrils is their effect upon the nervous system. In the process of investigating the human body/breath linkage as a context for self-unfoldment, the yogis discovered that there is a pattern of nostril dominance. They noticed that the nostrils progressed through a cycle whereby either the

* O'Brien, Justin, *Running and Breathing,* (Lakemont, GA: CSA Press, 1985) 38.

right or left nostril would flow predominantly while the other would decrease in air flow. They observed that this cycle lasted about one hour and fifty minutes in a healthy individual, and would automatically reverse after that time elapsed. They also observed that the nostrils would change to meet certain conditions. For instance, after eating, the right nostril would open, and when one was thirsty the left would predominate. When one was active or aggressive the right nostril would flow freely; when one was reflective or depressed, the left would open. At a few times during the day both nostrils are equally open for a brief time. This phenomenon is associated with a peaceful, joyous state of mind due to the perfect balance of the air flow. The yogis catalogued many such correlations and worked out methods for controlling the emotions and bodily functions by controlling the breath through the rhythm of nostril dominance. Today this rhythm is referred to as the infradian rhythm.*

Dr. O'Brien noticed this shift of nostril dominance during exercise, and says that,

> Running tends to produce either of the following two breath dominances: Usually the right nostril flares open during the run, associating with the vigorous activity; but there are moments when both nostrils sustain the force of air simultaneously. . . . Running does not produce left nostril breathing. Even when the left side may have been dominant at the beginning of the workout, the body quickly alters the breath flow to the right side or to the middle state.†

*See Swami Rama,   et al., *Yoga and Psychotherapy*, (Honesdale: PA. Himalayan Press, 1976) Ch. 2 for more information on breath rhythms.
† O'Brien, op. cit., 40.

The layers of lining in the nasal passages are partly responsible for the physiology of the rhythm of breathing. The mucous lining which moistens and cleans is in direct contact with the incoming air. Underneath the mucous lining we find a venus plexus which heats or cools the incoming air and also serves to engorge the erectile tissue located there. This tissue expands and contracts depending upon which nostril is engorged with blood at any specific moment. If you look up the nasal passage in a mirror, you will see how the tissues of the open and closed nostrils look.

The yogis developed a system of techniques to control nostril dominance. Through *swara yoga* (the yoga of breath) they were able to demonstrate significant impact on the function of the body and mind through the manipulation of the nostrils. They gained access to autonomic functions in part through manipulating nostril dominance and breath rhythms. The genius of impacting autonomic functioning through the vehicle of the breath can be appreciated when we realize that the breath is under both voluntary and involuntary control. By being able to consciously interface with the involuntary branches of the nervous system, yogis are able to gain subjective access to portions of unconscious patterns of behavior. In so doing they are able to subject autonomic behavior to stimulation and experimentation, or suppress it altogether.*

Science is becoming more aware of the breathing rhythms and is adding the proof of modern technology

* For full documentation on the experiments with yogi Swami Rama at the Menninger Foundation, see *The World Book Science Annual, 1974,* (Chicago: Field Enterprises Educational Corporation) 137-146.

to the knowledge that yogic sages discovered through critical self-observation. In *Science of Breath* Dr. Rudolph Ballentine states, in his section on nasal functioning of the limbic system,

> Neurophysiologists have found that inhalation not only stimulates the olfactory nerve when the air contains substances that can be sensed with the sense of smell, it also triggers neuronal messages in the olfactory nerve even when the air is clean. Why this occurs is not known. It is known, however, that the olfactory nerve and the part of the brain that it reaches is integrally connected to the limbic system, that part of the central nervous system which subserves emotional states.*

In an article in *Psychology Today* David Shannahoff Khalsa reported on experiments that were able to electronically validate what the yogis subjectively unravelled. They found that nasal cycles correspond to brain hemisphere cycles as indicated by EEG activity. They also found that in all subjects studied they could manipulate hemispherical dominance of the brain through forcibly closing one nostril.† Thus it seems that the infradian rhythm which affects, or is affected by, hemispherical dominance, greatly influences the way we see the world.

Let us now examine the types of breathing. For teaching it is helpful to break the breath down into categories or types based on the physiology implemented and the emotional response patterns stimulated. Paradoxical breathing is not a natural part of the breath cycle, but is rather dysfunctional breathing. Because

---

* Swami Rama et al., *Science of Breath*, 87.

† David Shannahoff Khalsa, "Rhythms and Reality: The Dynamics of Mind" in *Psychology Today*, September, 1984, 72-73.

it is observed so frequently, however, I include it here
for study.

Diaphragmatic Breathing

Diaphragmatic breathing occurs when the diaphragm
is used primarily for breathing. As we have seen, the
chest cavity is sealed and its internal pressure (pounds
per square inch) in the relaxed position equals that of
the outside atmosphere. When relaxed, the diaphragm
is in a domed position of exhalation, and for inhalation
it is contracted or flattened. This increases the volume
of the chest cavity but decreases its internal pressure.

Nature seeks to equalize differences of pressure. The
inhalation cycle of breathing occurs when gasses from
the atmosphere rush in through the nostrils, down the
trachea into the lungs to equalize the now decreased
pressure in the chest cavity. The exhalation cycle occurs
when the elastic recoil of the lung tissue, diaphragm,
and rib cage compress upon the inhaled gas. This then
increases the pressure in the chest cavity causing it to
be greater than that of the atmosphere. Obeying
nature's law, the gasses in the lungs then rush out into
the atmosphere in order to create a balance between
atmosphere and chest pressure once again. This cycle of
contraction of the diaphragm, decrease of pressure,
inrushing gas, elastic recoil, increase of pressure, out-
rush of gas is the basic cycle that the human body
uses for breathing.

The body was designed for diaphragmatic breathing.
This is supported in part through the construction of
the lungs, blood flow, and gravity. The heart pumps
waste-laden blood through the lungs in order for the
blood cells to give up carbon dioxide gasses and other

toxins into the lungs for exhalation. The heart pumps each blood cell single file through the capillaries, which are passing through the air sacks in the lungs. The process of respiration is the exchange in the red blood cell of waste products for oxygen.

Due to gravity the largest quantity of blood passing through the lungs for this exchange of oxygen occurs in the lower portion of the lobes of the lungs. Diaphragmatic breathing is the only way that the breath can be drawn fully into the bottom of the lungs. Thoracic and clavical breathing uses only the middle or upper portion of the lungs. When these latter two breaths are used exclusively, the heart is required to pump much more blood per minute through the lungs in order to satisfy the oxygen needs of the system. This causes undue strain on the heart over a period of years, and can contribute to dysfunction of the heart.

Although diaphragmatic breathing is the way nature intended us to breathe, most people, by the time they have physically matured, have interfered with this natural breath cycle. Thus diaphragmatic breathing must be relearned. In my work I have noticed that many clients find it difficult to consciously direct diaphragmatic movement correctly. Since abdominal breathing, which is much easier to consciously perform, promotes diaphragmatic breathing, I teach this easier method initially to beginners.

Abdominal Breathing

Abdominal breathing occurs when the breath cycle is generated from abdominal movement. As explained earlier, the abdomen is an airtight cavity and shares the diaphragm as a common partition with the chest cavity.

Like that in the chest cavity, the pressure in the abdomen is the same as that in the atmosphere. When the
abdominal muscles are distended, the volume of the
abdominal cavity increases, thus lowering its internal
pressure. In seeking to equalize the pressure in the
abdomen, the walls of the cavity are drawn in upon
themselves, and the diaphragm, which is the only other
flexible part of the system, is drawn down in order to
take up the displaced area, thus keeping the pressure
equalized in the abdominal cavity. We now have a
displacement in the chest cavity at the diaphragm which
meets the conditions for inhalation. Then the elastic
recoil present in the lungs, ribs, and diaphragm, along
with the contracting of the abdominal muscles, causes
the abdomen to return to its resting position. This
increases the pressure in the abdomen and contributes
to the increase of pressure in the chest, causing exhalation to take place so that the pressure in these two
cavities decreases to equal that of the outside atmosphere.

Because the abdominal muscles are so easily under
conscious control, it is quite simple to teach the
manipulation of the diaphragm via the abdomen to
beginning students. Once this is mastered direct access
to the diaphragm can be explored.

Thoracic Breathing

Thoracic breathing occurs when the muscles between the ribs are used to expand the ribcage, and thus
the lungs. The ribcage is expanded out and up because
of the directions of influence that the two layers of
intercostal muscles have upon the ribs. This type of
breathing is designed by nature to augment normal

diaphragmatic and abdominal breathing cycles. Thoracic breathing is employed in the case of emergency or in situations of greater oxygen needs (such as physical exertion or fear) for a greater expansion of the lungs.

Clavical Breathing

Breathing with the collar bones and upper chest is called clavical breathing. It is achieved through a raising of the shoulders and upper chest cavity which exerts a pull on the lungs from the top. The displacement is very little, and thus only a small quantity of oxygen is drawn into the system. My experience has been that this type of breathing is associated with stress and creates anxiety.

Paradoxical Breathing

I mention paradoxical breathing here not because it is a natural form of breathing but because it is a pattern of breathing associated with stress that is often used by many people. In breathing paradoxically the abdomen is contracted on the inhalation pressing the diaphragm up. This is the usual exhalation movement for both the abdomen and the diaphragm. Such movement forces the inhalation up into the rib cage and shoulders (intercostal and clavical breathing). Typically paradoxical breathing is employed at times of stress when the oxygen requirements are greater. Mechanically, however, the amount of oxygen drawn into the system is less because only the middle and upper portions of the lobes are being moved. This requires that the heart beat faster in order to oxygenate the blood properly, thus putting undue stress upon the heart.

In correct breathing the diaphragm is the primary source of movement for the expansion and contraction of the lungs and the transport of gas. This movement also provides valuable stimulation for the digestive and eliminative systems. The liver particularly is very dependent upon the diaphragm for its physical movement, and if the diaphragm is frozen or moved only slightly, liver function decreases in efficiency. The intestines also receive valuable stimulation from the pressure put on the abdominal cavity from diaphragmatic and/or abdominal muscular movement. The heart likewise receives massage from the motion of the diaphragm with each breathing cycle. When one breathes dysfunctionally, i.e., exclusive thoracic or clavical breathing, and immobilizes the diaphragm and abdomen, this important stimulation to digestion, elimination, and circulation is decreased, if not eliminated.

In terms of the autonomic nervous system, sympathetic and parasympathetic functioning is linked to breathing. When one breathes abdominally, one stimulates the parasympathetic nervous system, promoting the ongoing maintenance of the body system in general and generating a sense of ease and relaxation. When one breathes intercostally or thoracically one stimulates the sympathetic nervous system and signals to the brain that more energy is needed to cope with an impending emergency. This takes the body into a state of excitation, which, if unregulated and maintained for a prolonged period of time, creates an experience of stress and anxiety in the organism.

Here we find the therapeutic application for breathing properly. Chronic dysfunctional breathing puts the nervous system in a state of unresolved alarm. The hormones that are secreted into the blood stream as a result of this alarm alter one's thinking. This shift predisposes one to draw upon defensive or fear-oriented experiences from the memory reserves in the brain. One is then functioning with a nervous system motivated out of a sense of emergency rather than a nervous system motivated out of a sense of its own harmony and ease. It is not that arousal is improper for the system to experience; the nervous system is designed to be stimulated to high states of arousal. It is rather the prolonged, unregulated arousal that creates dysfunction in the system and promotes thought patterns motivated out of emotional pressure. Decreasing or eliminating the opportunity to interact with the current event on its own merit causes one to become firmly enmeshed in historical patterns of anxiety and sensations of being ill at ease.

The human organism is not designed to be in a parasympathetic mode at all times. There is a creative give and take between the two systems that generates balance for the organism. It is important to allow a natural rhythm of sympathetic and parasympathetic cycles in the body.* In fact, excessive parasympathetic stimulation can take an individual into an experience of depression. I have found that clients who are prone towards physical difficulties such as asthma or excessive sleep tend into a stress pattern referred to by Dr. Phil Nuernberger in *Freedom From Stress* as the possum effect.† The type of individual who employs

---

* For further information on this rhythm cycle see the *Research Bulletins* of the Himalayan Institute Dana Laboratory.

† Phil Nuernberger, Ph.D., op. cit., p. 69.

this strategy to encounter difficulty tends to repress emotions. The one who employs respiratory dysfunctions turns the emotion upon himself; the one who employs sleep as a strategy attempts to escape by going unconscious.

The exclusive use of the emergency nervous system through the breath (intercostal, clavical, and paradoxical breathing) during everyday functioning disrupts the rhythms of the breath and nervous system and has an adverse psychological impact upon the personality. This exclusive and inappropriate stimulation of the nervous system is the equivalent of using a S.W.A.T. team to watch over the behavior of a kindergarten class. This inappropriate use is a reflection of confused thinking and mobilization of resources.

The breath and body are so closely linked that while seeking to provide an environment for transformation, transformation in one will be reflected in the other. This is held to be true to the extent that we include the breath as an essential element for personal development in our holistic model.

Using the vocabulary of the breath as a therapeutic tool will give one immediate insight into the source of emotions. There will always be a corresponding shift in breath and body when there is an emotional shift. If the breath is used to hold back emotional experience, it is valuable to employ breathing practices so that the body may return to a state that allows for the experiencing of life as it is. By regulating the movement of the breath through the nostrils, the lungs, the diaphragm, one's neck (and thus the face) will be released, taking pressure off the skull, which will begin to generate an overall feeling of physical serenity.

Of the many yogic techniques practiced, two are especially useful in releasing physical tension and stress in the body. Swami Rama mentions that "Alternate nostril breathing has been found very useful in dealing with nervous disorders and deep, even breathing can help in relaxing tension." * He then gives four basic qualities to watch for in proper breathing. These are breathing deeply, so that the full lung capacity is used, eliminating any pause between inhalation and exhalation, breathing smoothly, and breathing without any sound.

The breathing technology developed by the yogis from the results of their experiments, though designed for inner exploration, has high therapeutic value. Listed here are specific breathing techniques that are found to be very useful for therapeutic intervention.

> Abdominal breathing
> Diaphragmatic breathing
> Even breathing
> Complete breath
> Bellows breathing
> Alternate nostril breathing
> Breathing for sleep

The first four techniques are best learned lying on the back. This is so because when one lies on the back nature automatically shifts the breathing into the diaphragm or abdomen unless the breathing is severely paradoxical.

We are giving the breath as an object of concentration in order to eliminate emotional involvement

*Swami Rama, op.cit., 25, 27.

with internal dialogue. The intent here is to bring the client into the present, which will reduce emotional involvement in regards to historical responses to the current upset or stimulation. This is true for all the breathing practices.

ABDOMINAL BREATHING

Technique: Lie on your back. Place your right hand on your abdomen, left hand on your chest. The right hand should move and the left hand should not. When you exhale, the right hand should go down, and when you inhale the right hand should rise.

Points to Notice: Be sure that you are breathing smoothly, with no pauses, jerks, or sound, and that the breath is moving through the nostrils. Do not strain. Let your exhalation and your inhalation be equal. Emotional involvement with internal dialogue should be eliminated.

Purpose: This is a valuable technique to initially work with the breath because the abdominal muscle is very easily put under conscious control. When one breathes abdominally, one breathes diaphragmatically. This technique is not necessarily designed to be used for the whole of one's life. Diaphragmatic breathing is the type of breath that nature designed our body to use. When you want to bring a dramatic relaxation response to the system, utilize abdominal breathing and it will draw you very quickly into a deeper state of relaxation. Abdominal breathing is also very valuable for reconnecting individuals who are estranged from their body, e.g., those disassociated from survival, sexuality, and power urges.

DIAPHRAGMATIC BREATHING

This exercise can be done either seated or lying down. It is much easier, however, to learn it lying down on your back. In this breathing the diaphragm is the primary source of movement. As a result there will not be very much abdominal or intercostal movement. I recommend this method as a goal for one's normal breathing process.

Technique: Place the right hand on the abdomen at the navel or below, and the left hand on the chest. While breathing neither hand should move appreciably. The section between the two hands should move. This area between the sternum and the navel will move up and down with the inhalation and exhalation respectively while the lower ribs will move out and in.

You can assist yourself in learning this exercise with the two following techniques. First, take a three pound sandbag and place it on the abdomen between the sternum and the navel. With the hands placed on the lower abdomen and chest, cause the sandbag to rise and fall with each breath. Be sure that the bag rises on the inhalation and falls on the exhalation. This will assure you that you are not breathing paradoxically. Second, take the two hands and place them on the lower rib cage at the floating ribs. Each time you inhale, your hands will be pushed outwards with the expansion of the ribs, and each time you exhale, your hands will move back in. This movement is a reflection of the motion of the diaphragm and its impact upon the ribcage. At some point you will be able to breathe diaphragmatically with no aids whatsoever.

Points to Notice: Be sure that you are not breathing paradoxically. Be sure that you are breathing smoothly, with no pauses, jerks, or sound, and that the breath is moving through the nostrils. Do not strain. Let your exhalation and your inhalation be equal. Emotional involvement with internal dialogue should be eliminated.

Purpose: This exercise is valuable because it teaches the kind of breath that nature intended. It has access to the sympathetic and parasympathetic stimulation, and allows one access to the energies and behaviors associated with each.

EVEN BREATHING

Technique: This technique is best learned lying on the floor. Abdominal or diaphragmatic breathing is to be used. In this technique exhalation and inhalation will be of equal length and done through the nostrils. Explore to determine the length of exhalation and inhalation that lies within your capacity without straining. Once you have determined this, gradually, over a period of weeks or months, increase the length of each breath to the point where you will be able to exhale for fifteen seconds and inhale for fifteen seconds with ease. Start with five minutes of practice and work up to fifteen minutes.

Variation: If a person is distraught and is becoming over-emotional, have him lie down on his front in the crocodile pose (see p. 209) and perform even breathing.

This will slow the breathing down because of the body weight on the abdomen and diaphragm. The slower breath rhythms will change the emotional state, and will also automatically cause diaphragmatic breathing to be implemented.

Points to Notice: Take specific care to allow no pause between either the exhalation and inhalation, or the inhalation and exhalation. Be sure that you are breathing smoothly, with no pauses, jerks, or sound, and that the breath is moving through the nostrils. Do not strain. Let your exhalation and your inhalation be equal. Emotional involvement with internal dialogue should be eliminated.

Purpose: There are a number of therapeutic values in this exercise, one of which is to stimulate the relaxation rebound for the nervous system. This technique reduces stress and so can be used at the end of the day to assist the nervous system to return to normalcy. The reason I point out this value is that some problems cannot be resolved in the course of the day. However, the nervous system must be allowed to go to a state of ease so that living can go on as the problems persist. This technique creates the environment for that to happen, allowing the nervous system to be restimulated when the situation or problem arises again.

COMPLETE BREATH

This breath utilizes the entire breathing mechanism from the abdomen up to the shoulders. It is a special breathing technique and is not to be employed excessively or indiscriminately.

Technique: The complete breath can be done both lying down and sitting up, but is best learned lying down. Exhale completely, then begin inhaling with the abdomen. Keep on inhaling with the diaphragm, in the middle chest, continue inhaling by expanding your back, ending by expanding the upper chest. This should be done without any strain or holding of breath. Then exhale by contracting the abdominal muscles and then slowly compressing the chest from the diaphragm up to the collarbone.

Variation: In an advanced application of this breathing technique, rather than having the exhalation and inhalation equal, have the exhalation twice as long as the inhalation. It has been noted by the research laboratories at the Himalayan Institute that the exhalation is part of the parasympathetic response system, and as a result, relaxation rebound is stimulated to a larger extent when the exhalation is twice as long as the inhalation.

Points to Notice: Be sure that you are breathing smoothly, with no pauses, jerks, or sound, and that the breath is moving through the nostrils. Do not strain. Let your exhalation and your inhalation be equal. Emotional involvement with internal dialogue should eliminated. Be sure that you discriminate and expand your breathing mechanism piece by piece to ensure maximum and full expansion of the lungs.

Purpose: This breathing technique most definitely brings about a feeling of well-being and can be used as a preface to meditation.

BELLOWS BREATHING

This technique is used as a preliminary to the alternate nostril breathing exercise.

Technique: Sit with your head, neck, and trunk erect. Actively and sharply contract your abdominal muscles so as to forcibly cause the exhalation to take place. Then relax the abdominal muscles, letting them move to their normal position which will passively allow an inhalation to take place. Let us say, for example, that it took you one-quarter second to exhale, then the recoil might naturally use three-quarters of a second. Thus your cycle would be one breath rhythm per second. Repeat this movement of contraction and relaxation rhythmically and continue it eleven to twenty-one times in the beginning, eventually expanding up to one minute.

Caution: If you have high blood pressure, heart problems, epilepsy, or severe asthma, do not use this technique, but consider the complete breath in its stead.

Points to Notice: Be sure that you are breathing abdominally and not paradoxically. The breath should be passing through your nostrils, and there should be no sounds coming from your throat. The throat is to be maintained as relaxed as possible. If there is any sound such as wheezing, ease up on the vigor of your breathing so as not to cause any damage to your respiratory system.

Purpose: Bellows breathing is a grosser cleansing technique than alternate nostril breathing with the intention to somewhat radically impact the entire physiology with the breath through aggressive, rapid breathing.

ALTERNATE NOSTRIL BREATHING

As we have ascertained, at any given time the breath flows more through one nostril than another. Alternate nostril breathing manipulates this rhythm of nostril dominance. Exhalation and inhalation in this exercise are to be equal. Start with a breath length that is very comfortable for you and gradually work up to a fifteen second exhalation and a fifteen second inhalation. Give yourself the weeks or months necessary to arrive at this duration comfortably.

Technique: Find the nostril that flows the easiest. From here on it will be referred to as the active nostril. The one that does not flow as easily will be referred to as the passive nostril. If both nostrils are flowing equally then choose one to be the active. This technique is not to be done while lying down.

Sit with your head, neck, and torso erect, either in a chair or on the floor, using the following gesture with your right hand. Curl the index and middle fingers in, placing them on the palm of the hand. This will leave your thumb, ring, and small fingers extended. Place the thumb at the right nostril and the ring finger at the left nostril. Close your passive nostril without moving the cartilege of the nose, and slowly, gently, and subtly exhale, using the complete breath through the active nostril, for a specific period of time. Close the active nostril and inhale through the passive nostril for the same period of time. Continue breathing this way using the following pattern:

1. Exhale active	2. Inhale passive
3. Exhale active	4. Inhale passive
5. Exhale active	6. Inhale passive
7. Exhale passive	8. Inhale active
9. Exhale passive	10. Inhale active
11. Exhale passive	12. Inhale active

Lower your hands to your lap and be aware of the breath as it spontaneously passes through your nostrils. At some point you will be able to control nostril dominance mentally and will not have to use your hand.

Points to Notice: Be sure that the spine remains erect and that you are putting no strain on your nose or pressing it off center. Be sure that you are breathing smoothly, with no pauses, jerks, or sound, and that the breath is moving through the nostrils. Do not strain. Let your exhalation and your inhalation be equal. Emotional involvement with internal dialogue should be eliminated.

Purpose: This technique, according to the yogis, strengthens the nervous system's capacity to tolerate emotional stimulation. I utilize this method as a means to increase the client's ability to be involved with life without becoming emotionally dysfunctional. This allows him then to utilize the training and insight he has received while involved in any emotionally-charged situation. This technique increases the probability of him acting out of his wisdom rather than acting out of his anticipation and conditioning.

BREATHING FOR SLEEP

This technique is given for those who have difficulty falling asleep at night.

Technique: Lie on your left side. Count twenty-one exhalations and inhalations as they occur. This will open your right nostril. Then roll over unto your right side. Again count twenty-one exhalations and inhalations. This will open your left nostril. Next lie on your back and exhale and inhale twenty-one times. You should be asleep by now. If not, do this cycle twice more.

Points to Notice: Be aware that you are breathing abdominally with no strain. The intention here is not to breathe to your capacity, but just to count the breaths that go by naturally.

Purpose: The intent here is to bring the mind into the present and take it off distracting thoughts. The yogis found that this rhythm of right nostril, left nostril, both nostrils tends to induce the experience of sleep in the practitioner.

12
Meditation

Self-discovery has been a pursuit of humankind since its existence. We have as a species continually sought, in many ways, a communication with, and an understanding of, ourselves. In seeking to fathom our origins, we have sought a natural and logical unfoldment of our minds. The ancient sages and seers of every culture likewise followed this pursuit. Yogic sages codified their experiments in this seeking and passed them on to those who would follow.

It is this bank of knowledge, based on experience that has been tried, tested, and proved for centuries that we offer here. These are preliminary and very basic techniques that are the foundation of self-discovery from the perspective of the yogic sages. In inventing this program, they sought to assist aspirants in unlocking the treasure within by making repressed and unintelligible dimensions of the mind visible. A subtle and very powerful therapy was devised by them for this purpose. They knew that it was essential for the aspirants' involvement to be with life as it is, that learning could take place only when the aspirants are no longer possessed by the need to protect what they had become.

We are very like Theseus going through the labyrinth to the Minotaur in the center. The many who had gone before him got lost in the convoluted corridors of the maze. None of the passages led to the center, but were an end unto themselves. The sages sought to expose the various emotional behaviors that we create as a labyrinth in our mind. They used meditation as the thread that leads through these corridors to the very center of being.

Self-discovery is the place where yoga and modern therapy interface. The tools of meditation gathered by the yogic sages lend themselves very admirably to the achievement of therapeutic intervention. The therapist is seeking to coach the client in self-knowledge and the expansion of choices. Doing this without imposing his own set of limits requires a subtlety and vigilence that escapes almost all of us.

What is necessary, then, is to create a physical and mental environment that will be conducive for the exploration and harmonizing of the maze of emotions within. When one takes time for meditation, one moves towards an environment where the existence of self-discovery can appear. It is a gradual process of penetrating through one's self-defenses. Following is a brief outline of the classical approach to this end.

First it is important to cultivate a mental attitude which is open to the insights meditation will provide. The *yamas* and *niyamas* are some suggested guidelines for cultivating this attitude. Equally important is finding a posture where the head, neck, and torso can be erect and comfortable during the practice so that the body does not create a disturbance for the other parts of the mind during this exploration. This is done also to provide ease of energy flow, such as unimpaired breathing and blood circulation, as well as energy passage through the spine. Next, the nervous system must be put at ease so as not to toss one's awareness around like the proverbial fish on the sea of emotions spoken of earlier. Breathing exercises are primarily utilized to accomplish this emotional ease. In moving closer toward the meditative state, one's sensual interest in the ongoing rush of external phenomenon is attenuated. Progressive relaxation exercises are used at this point to withdraw one's awareness from continued involvement with sensory objects which would encourage continued excitation. Next, concentration is created by the use of a focusing object that has the capacity to lead the meditator to the silence within. Meditation is sitting in that silence and maintaining the concentration in a pure, unalloyed form for an extended period of time. Finally, meditation deepens into the state of *samadhi*. In this state, no questions remain. In a very real manner one's own self is realized as the self of all.

The Ontology of Meditation

Technically speaking, meditation is a state wherein the meditator is able to hold an object fixedly within his awareness without deviation. As meditation deepens, the distinction between the object and the meditator begins to diminish. Eventually there is complete assimilation of the object by the subject to the point where the two no longer exist as separate, but show up as one, meditating. The arrival at this point is called *samadhi*, which is the essential technique of yoga.

The use of this technique of *samadhi* is applied to the assimilation and transcendence of the levels and grades of one's being. For the yogis, the eventual goal of life is to be liberated from unconscious participation with the paradigm called "becoming." It is said by them that the achievement of this liberation establishes one as the paradigm of paradigms. This paradigm that creates all other paradigms is called the essential self— Existence. While this unfoldment is taking place, techniques of meditation and *samadhi* are applied to explore the paradigm of "becoming."

The yogic sages experienced how the mind becomes its environment. When the mind creates an ego (in other words, a perspective), the ego becomes identified with its own creation. This is the power of the mind. As we have seen, it has the ability to become whatever it sets itself to, be it human, ecstatic, attracted, repulsed, female, aged, disappointed, or whatever. The sages were clear that the paradigm called "being" is the true illuminator of the mind and that "becoming" mind comes into existence by the ability to make distinctions. Mind illumined by being "becomes" the distinctions it makes. This is a reflection of being. The

intelligence to be responsible for making those distinctions empowers the individual to assimilate,
transcend, and thus tap what he has become. Thus
enlightened, the yogis empowered themselves at one
level as the creators, and transcending that, they became
liberated from the paradigm called mind.

We see the vital point in human development as
letting go of attachment to what one has so essentially
and skillfully become. In so doing, one remains free to
employ that strategy of behavior, while at the same time
involving himself in a learning mode with other behaviors that he will eventually become. Becoming, then,
is the provision of a context for learning to take place.
Becoming confines one's view in order to gain a perspective on life. Once the perspective has been organized
and invested with selfhood, that is, one now exclusively
becomes its perspective, the next step is to release oneself from the exclusivity.

My experience has been that this exclusivity can be
released only when we assuage our fear of annihilation
by letting go of our attachment to what we have
become. In the process of unfolding the potentials
within our being, we assimilate life through becoming
it. In the sense that we think we are what we have
become, we experience the fear associated with change.
It is important for us to realize in full confidence that
the various levels of our ego, once awakened, will never
be destroyed. The self of being has awakened to each
level of ego by becoming it. These levels of ego are,
as it were, immortalized in a transcendent self. We no
longer exclusively identify ourself with one particular
becoming, one particular I, who is the living learning
phase. We are in a transpersonal phase; all of it is in us,

but all of us is not in it. Consequently, there is no annihilation taking place. There is the opportunity now to choose from a vast pool of actualized being that previously had been a boundary line of self-identification. This is another way to say *samadhi*, for it is the transcendental, intelligent, absolute becoming.

Therapeutic Application of Meditation

In a therapeutic setting the techniques and basic applications of preliminary meditation can be applied very simply to initiate a climate for self-observation. Meditation can assist individual clients in achieving conscious access to their dream states and subconscious material. As we have seen, the storage of historical decisions has a very strong impact upon our present-based behavior. When sitting in meditation the scenarios that act themselves out will be motivated from historical and emotional intent which is sometimes confused as one's own internal dialogue. Perhaps it is not one thinking at all, but merely "thinking" taking place.

During meditation we see the parade of images and/or feel the sensations that normally pass outside of awareness. One of the essential keys to self-observation is to let all of this take place without becoming disturbed by it. After having achieved a settling of the nervous system into a state of ease, we learn to sit and witness, as it were, the passage of this internal dialogue.

The difficulty that arises in meditation practice, however, is that we begin to brood upon the memories that come forward. We then attempt to mentally manipulate these memories to come out a certain way. Depending upon our success or lack of it, due to the context of our interpretation, we will have emotional reactions to these memories. From a yogic viewpoint there is a paradigm that describes this process of brooding.

> As a person broods on the objects of the senses, there arises in him attachment to them; from attachment arises desire; from thwarted desire anger is produced. From anger comes delusion; from delusion, the confusion of memory and loss of mindfulness; from the disappearance of memory and mindfulness, the loss of the faculty of discrimination; by loss of the faculty of discrimination, one perishes.
>
> Bhagavad Gita, II. 62-63

If one constantly broods on an event or experience, one will become attached to his interpretation of it and the need for future events to come to the same conclusion. If this expectation is thwarted he will become frustrated. According to Swami Rama,

> That frustration leads to anger toward that which is frustrating him. Unfulfilled desire or dissatisfaction is thus the cause of anger. When one becomes angry, he forgets to use discrimination and his memory wavers. That leads to the loss of reason, and one's mind becomes completely imbalanced.*

Here again we can appreciate the insight of the sages. They have created a technique for an individual to be "on purpose" while in a dimension of the mind usually out of conscious awareness.

In meditation one most definitely travels through the behavioral side of the mind typically associated with dreams. This is where much of human behavior lives. The structure of one's other-than-conscious strategies

---

*Swami Rama, *Perennial Psychology of the Bhagavad Gita*, (Honesdale, PA: Himalayan Press, 1985) 110.

of behavior is constantly articulating itself outside of awareness. It is like Rumpelstiltskin (our other-than-conscious strategies) who, while in the forest (the terrain of the other-than-conscious mind), unfolded the truth about himself by saying his name (his nature). This was easily heard by the agent (one's awareness) sent by the queen (one's self in meditation).

As a result of being awake in the daydreaming state, much about oneself can be learned. For example, when you realize that these things just take place and begin to explore the fact that your responses are a historical you, your options of behavior begin to expand. You come to realize that you have some additional choices, and that in the past you made some decisions that defined who you were. This definition gave you a perspective from which to view the world. Now that perspective persists. It is no longer you who wakes up in the morning, but your history that rolls out of bed. As a result of that, any event that takes place before you ends up being acted upon by your history. Your choices are stored in your interpretation or what you say about it, for what you say is for you what it is.

Meditation teaches one, among many other things, to choose one's interaction with life. It does so initially by letting one interact with the dream state while awake, and at the same time teaching one how to be undisturbed by what comes up out of the mind. One will come to know that what is there is there, and one can be uneffected by it.

Our thought process happens in large part on an other-than-conscious level. As with the body, so through thoughts or language, one can impact behavior on a rational and non-rational level. We have an image of ourself within. Who we think we are is stored in this self-concept. We then end up living out of this interpretation of ourself. We have many memories filed that support this self-image, and when an event in life interfaces with it we act in ways to protect and maintain that self-image. We then translate, through language, our interpretation of this interface, and we live through our translation of it.

Remember the belief cycle that was outlined in chapter five? What we believe we expect, what we expect we observe, what we observe reinforces our belief. What we find ourself doing is reorganzing our experience of an event to fit within our interpretation of that event. We will literally cut out pieces of data that are not congruent with our interpretation of life. In so doing we live in a world of rationalized construction, lessening the opportunity to live with what is.

Piaget, the renowned scientist who studied learning theory, speaks of this selecting out and changing that occurs in human behavior. Part of his proposal is that knowledge is not a copy of reality, but a construction of reality, and when we are mistaken, we are systematically mistaken. In being a construction, knowledge and input are not identical.*

This is demonstrated in part by an experiment conducted by Michael Cole in 1973. He selected a group of African hunters and arranged models of an antelope, a rhinoceros, and a hunter holding a gun on a sheet of paper before them individually. For half of the Africans

*Herb Koplowicz, "Piaget's Constructionist Epistemology," unpublished paper, 11.

he placed the model of the rhinoceros in the upper left hand corner of the paper, and in all of the cases he placed the hunter in the lower left hand corner with the rifle aimed up at the upper left corner. The antelope was placed in the upper right hand corner in all cases (fig. 1). For the other half of the Africans he placed nothing in the upper left hand corner of the paper, while the other two figures were placed the same as before (fig.2). Time was allowed to elapse and all participants were then requested to arrange the models themselves the way they had been shown. The first group, which had been shown the hunter in the lower left with the rifle pointed to the rhinoceros in the upper left corner (fig. 1) reassembled the models accurately. The second group, which did not have the rhinoceros in the upper left corner, more often than not pointed the rifle at the antelope in the upper right hand corner (fig. 3).*

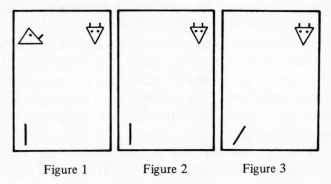

Figure 1   Figure 2   Figure 3

It is apparent that the African hunters thought it senseless for the hunter to be pointing a gun in a direction away from the target, and so they changed the

* Cole, Michael, *Culture and Thought* (New York: Wiley, 1974).

placement of the figures to correspond with their construction, or "map," of reality. What is true was at dissonance with what they knew. It is apparent how this supports Piaget's structure of knowledge, and also apparent how valuable this is for us in life.

I use this example to support the therapeutic relevance of meditation. This is the circumstance in which we find ourselves organizing reality. We live according to our interpretation or "map" of our reality.

The therapeutic value of meditation lies in its invitation to let life come without reference to, or dependence upon, any presuppositions that one may hold. It enhances the opportunity to experience life as it is, because one is not imposing history on the present. Having a history is very valuable, but one must be free to choose the consulting view given by that history. It is like Aunt Agnes. Her advice can be noteworthy as long as one can choose to consider her advice rather than letting her live in one's stead.

The sages designed the beginning steps of meditation to introduce the meditator to witness the constructions of reality that pass before his eyes and, by technique, encourage him not to become involved with what was taking place. This serves to assist the meditator in eventually seeing through his exclusive identification with his current construction of reality, and by witnessing, discharge the emotions associated with the construction.

What the technology of meditation brings forth is an opportunity to discharge emotions that logically connect different linguistic structures. With meditation we can make the mind a more comfortable place to be because we decrease the potency of an emotional logic makes the storage of past impressions frightful, guilt-ridden or any other behavior considered to be dysfunctional. An important point is making the mind a comfortable place to be. I find that this enhances therapeutic intervention and decreases the amount of time an individual needs to be in a therapeutic environment, because it gives him skills whereby he will be able to maintain a sense of equanimity without the need for anyone to intervene with him on his own behalf.

In making the mind a more comfortable place to be, we are acquainting, through the meditative process, the individual with the inner terrain of his mind. While meditating one is encouraged to remember the object of concentration. In so doing a sense of self-awareness can be maintained instead of investing selfhood in the memories that are encountered. If selfhood becomes invested in the memories, the thrust of meditation is lost because we now become the memories with all the emotion that ties the memories together.

Alice's pursuit of the White Rabbit in her adventures through Wonderland reminds me of this process. The rabbit is the object of concentration; the Mad Hatter and his tea party, the caterpiller, the flowers, and the Cheshire Cat are all qualities indigenous to the wonderland of the mind. They are merely a diversion when attention is invested in them. They are not intruders; they belong there. They are merely present along Alice's path. Alice's task is to follow the White Rabbit. She becomes diverted because of her inquiry which is based upon her construction of reality—her ego. She gives personal commentary about each feature with which she comes in contact.

We are doing the same thing as Alice when we

meditate if we listen to our internal dialogue, and if, in coming into contact with a piece of our history, we comment about it in attempts to manipulate it to fit our construction of reality, to make it the way we know it to be, like the African hunters. We need to meditate often in order to have the wide range of experience that Alice had. In this way we can learn through repetition how to creatively function in the wonderland of our mind, utilizing its inhabitants to point our way. We need to learn to relate to that hard-to-grasp Cheshire Cat with his beguiling smile and his "now you see me, now you don't" way of behaving. The terrain of the dream state is different from that of the waking state. We have the intelligence and power to tap the subconscious dream state as a resource and utilize its guidance.

In summary we point out the following therapeutic values which the model of meditation contains:

1. It creates an experience of meeting what is actually occurring.

2. It creates a willingness to be in the present, which is where life is taking place.

3. It puts perspective in perspective.

4. It can discharge the glue of emotional logic.

5. It instills a habit of listening to internal dialogue which will give a clue in daily life about one's belief structures.

6. It increases one's will power so that one is in a greater position to choose the present, thus putting together a string of successes based upon current choices or levels of wisdom.

BREATH AWARENESS MEDITATION

The following technique is an easily delivered and applied method of meditation that has the potential to bring forth all of the features that we have mentioned.

Technique: Sit with the head, neck, and trunk erect with the legs in a crossed position; or sit in a chair in the friendship pose. Imagine yourself surrounded by a comfortable, secure, self-presence. Do either Bellows Breath or Complete Breath to be followed by Alternate Nostril Breathing.

Then lower your hands to your lap and be aware of your abdominal movement which comes as a response to the breath. It is important not to consciously manipulate the breath or muscles. You are to be aware of the movement only. Let go of any presupposition about what a meditative breath is supposed to be.

After a period of time (of your own choosing) shift your awareness to the breath as it is flowing through your active nostril. Here your task is to be aware of whatever breath is already there. You are to refine the sensitivity of your awareness, not to make the breath grosser.

Next shift your awareness to the breath as it flows through the passive nostril. If there is no breath in the passive nostril, then be aware of the absence of breath. As you progress, nostril dominance will shift automatically for you through an act of quiet will.

After this bring your awareness to the breath at the point where the nostrils meet the upper lip, being aware of the breath flowing through both nostrils. Eventually they will flow in harmony and equilibrium. (This may take minutes or months.) When you achieve this harmony, there will be a most definite shift in sensorial experience, and a definite wave that you will interpret as joy will move through your system.

Spend the remainder of your meditation time attending to the breath passing through the nostrils while being undisturbed as you travel through the depths and breadth of your mind.

Sit for a time that is comfortable for you. It may vary from five minutes to an hour.

Come out slowly.

Points to Notice: Be aware of the breath passing through the nostrils. Do not force it. If you are not sensitive to the experience of the breath passing through the nostrils, allow the days, weeks, or months necessary for your awareness to become more refined. You may experience temperature, pressure, sound, images. Your role at this stage is to witness. It is important for you not to interpret the memories or phenomenon that will most assuredly appear. You, like Alice, are passing through an area replete with events. If you become involved you will add drama to these seeds, and they will sprout into full fantasy. Pass them by and follow the White Rabbit of your breath.

Purpose: This meditation will provide an environment whereby an increase in willingness to meet what is actually taking place and being in the present will become a greater part of one's daily life. This freedom unlocks our bondage to historical constructions of reality, frees us from historical choices that no longer serve us, unshackles us from living in a world of abstraction, and introduces us to the possibility of the wonder and surprise of a world that actually is.

Another and very vital purpose of this technique is to create a habit of observing the breath. This habit is to be carried on into daily life. The fruit of this habit is that upon remembering to experience the breath, you will also be aware of the last thought that went through your mind. This gives you periodic checks on your thought process. The breath as an object of concentration is so powerful because of its purity. The breath and its source exist with you on all levels and can be held as an object of concentration easier than most objects, without having to apply conscious effort. The breath can be followed to the center of the mind.

The quality of your breath has the capacity of itself to generate states of consciousness. The progressive breathing application of bellows, complete breath, breath awareness at abdomen, breath awareness at active nostril, breath awareness at passive nostril, and finally awareness of breath at the point where the nostrils meet the upper lip takes one from an overtly controlled breathing to more and more refined experiences of breathing. The technique of itself will guide you toward the center as the rabbit guided Alice through wonderland.

Below I list a process for an entire session from postures through meditation. Any one of the sections can also be done separately.

1. Relaxation

2. Postures

3. Relaxation

4. Breathing

    A. Bellows

    B. Alternate Nostril Breathing

        or

    C. Complete Breath

5. Breath Awareness Meditation